UNDERSTANDING HEART DISEASE

UNDERSTANDING HEART DISEASE

ARTHUR SELZER

UNIVERSITY OF CALIFORNIA PRESS
BERKELEY   LOS ANGELES   OXFORD

University of California Press
Berkeley and Los Angeles, California

University of California Press, Ltd.
Oxford, England

Library of Congress Cataloging-in-Publication Data

Selzer, Arthur.
    Understanding heart disease / Arthur Selzer.
        p.   cm.
    Includes index.
    ISBN 0-520-06560-3 (alk. paper)
        1. Heart—Diseases—Popular works.   I. Title.
RC672.S44   1992
616.1′2—dc20

                                                                92-4854

Printed in the United States of America
1   2   3   4   5   6   7   8   9

The paper used in this publication meets the minimum require-
ments of American National Standard for Information
Sciences—Permanence of Paper for Printed Library Materials,
ANSI Z39.48-1984. ⊗

Contents

Preface

This volume is the outgrowth of my book *The Heart: Its Function in Health and Disease,* originally published in 1966. In the nearly twenty-five years since that book first appeared, there has been extraordinary progress in the diagnosis and treatment of heart disease, along with a growth of public interest in and awareness of heart disease, which remains the number-one cause of death and disability despite a significant decline in the past few decades. In response to this high interest, the news media cover medical advances in the field of heart disease extensively. Exaggerated and premature reports of newer aspects of treatment frequently lead to misunderstanding and unreasonable expectations.

Along with the introduction of new technologies in the diagnosis and treatment of heart disease, there has been a growth in the number of hospitals and clinics providing specialized care for cardiac patients that is generally considered excessive. Furthermore, the question of whether too many complex diagnostic tests and operations are being performed on patients with heart disease has been raised and widely discussed in the news media and has aroused the interest of Congress. Among the reasons for this alleged overuse is the demand by the often poorly informed public for the "newest."

These considerations influenced me to shift the emphasis in this new book. Rather than update the previous volume, which discussed the normal and abnormal heart in simple terms, I decided to present the problems facing today's cardiologist, explaining the technologies and the decision-making process but avoiding direct advice to a cardiac patient—in other words, emphasizing the "why" rather than the "how" of prevention and treatment of heart disease. I hope that a better-informed reader in need of medical care will be able to cooperate more successfully with the physician.

To keep the book within the framework of these objectives, I eliminated certain subjects or discussed them only briefly. Among those are epidemiological data related to heart disease, such as statistics regarding the incidence, the age and sex, and the racial and geographical distribution of various types of heart disease. Similarly, I have omitted detailed presentations of treatment, including specific recommendations regarding drug and dietary management of heart disease, in favor of concise statements of principles.

Cardiologists now have a wide range of options, from conservative to aggressive, in managing patients. Many steps are subject to controversy and debate. In writing this book, I have attempted to take the middle-of-the-road attitude and identify controversial questions. The first two chapters review the structure and function of the normal heart and the circulation of blood. The following two chapters present general approaches to diagnosis and treatment of heart disease and describe the available technology. The balance of the book reviews the principal cardiac diseases, explaining their causes, recognition, and management.

Chapter One

The Normal Heart: Structure

General Definitions

The circulatory apparatus is a closed system filled with blood, consisting of the heart and blood vessels; it is the principal supply line between various organs and parts of the body. The circulation delivers fuel to the body, namely oxygen and other essential substances; it also removes carbon dioxide and other products of metabolism. Blood is circulated in two separate circuits: the smaller circuit is known as the *lesser circulation* or the *pulmonary circulation;* and the larger circuit, the *greater circulation* or the *systemic circulation.* The former supplies the lungs, the latter all other organs of the body. Figure 1 is a diagrammatic outline of the circulation, showing the lesser circulation above the heart and the greater circulation below the heart.

The central organ of the circulatory system is the *heart.* It consists of two separate pumps, one for each circuit, simultaneously ejecting an equal quantity of blood into the greater and the lesser circulation. The heart is a muscular organ weighing approximately 300 gm, which contracts rhythmically about 70 times a minute and with each beat expels about 75 cc of blood into each circuit. Each system of blood vessels into which the blood is pumped consists of three parts: the *arterial system*, the *capillary system*, and the *venous system*, as shown in figure 1. The objective of the lesser circulation is to send blood through the vessels of the lungs and there to bring it into close contact with the air, so that oxygen can

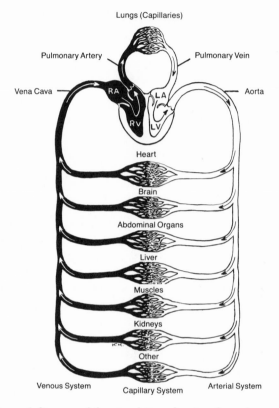

Figure 1. General diagram of the circulation showing the pulmonary circuit above the heart and the systemic circuit below the heart. Oxygenated blood is shown in white and deoxygenated blood in black.

be replenished and carbon dioxide removed; thus the blood in the pulmonary artery (leading to the lungs) has a low oxygen content and high carbon dioxide content, whereas blood returning from the lungs in the pulmonary veins has a high oxygen content and low carbon dioxide content. The objectives of the greater circulation are as follows: to deliver oxygen to the tissues; to pick up and deliver all nourishing substances, vitamins, hormones, and other vital compounds; to carry carbon dioxide, the "exhaust" of the tissues, to the right side of the heart and hence to the lungs for elimination; and to pick up other waste products and deliver them to the points of their excretion or elimination (kidneys, liver, etc.).

Oxygen is the most essential fuel for every tissue of the body. Its utilization is intimately connected with carbon dioxide, the principal waste product of tissues. Thus each cell in the body "breathes" by extracting oxygen from the blood and depositing carbon dioxide in its place. Blood destined for the tissues, fully saturated with oxygen and containing a lower quantity of carbon dioxide, is bright red. It is ordinarily referred to as *arterial blood,* as it is contained in the arteries of the greater circulation. Blood returning from the tissues has a lower oxygen content and is high in carbon dioxide; such blood, dark red in color, is termed *venous blood,* as it is contained in the veins of the greater circulation. It shines through the superficial veins under the skin, making them appear blue. It is clear from figure 1 that the terms "arterial blood" (indicated as white in the chart) and "venous blood" (indicated as black) apply only to the greater circulation. In the pulmonary circulation, as I have said, the role of arteries and veins is reversed. Figure 1 emphasizes the fact that the pulmonary circuit consists of a simple system of vessels supplying a single organ; the greater circulation, by contrast, consists of a great number of semiautonomous systems connected parallel to each other. Each organ of the body receives blood from arterial branches, which then divide into capillary branches. The actual exchange of all substances between the blood and tissues occurs within the capillary system.

Structure of the Heart

The heart is a muscular, conical organ located in the center of the chest, slightly more to the left than to the right (fig. 2). It has an apex, directed downward and leftward, and a base at its upper part where major vessels originate. The heart consists of three layers: an inner lining (*endocardium*); the heart muscle (*myocardium*); and the outer covering (*pericardium*). The pericardium itself has two layers: the outer lining of the heart (*epicardium*), which is firmly attached to it, giving the surface of the heart a smooth, glistening appearance; and a loose sac (*parietal pericardium*), in which the heart is suspended. This parietal pericardium is shown in figure 2, where the front portion of it has been removed in order to display details of the frontal aspect of the heart. Between the two layers of

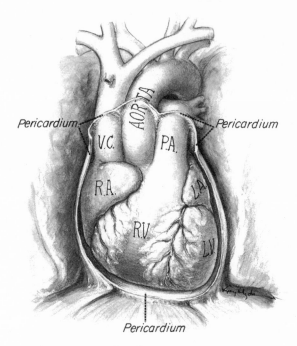

Figure 2. Frontal aspect of the heart with the parietal pericardium removed. Abbreviations: V.C. = superior vena cava; R.A. = right atrium; R.V. = right ventricle; P.A. = pulmonary artery.

the pericardium there is a small amount of fluid (*pericardial fluid*) which acts as a lubricant, facilitating motion of the heart within the pericardial sac.

The heart is a hollow organ comprising four chambers: two *atria* (the correct term "atrium" is often used interchangeably with the older term "auricle") and two *ventricles*. The thin-walled atria act as receptacles for the blood returning to the heart; the thick-walled ventricles, consisting of several layers of muscle, constitute the pump proper. The two atria and the two ventricles are separated from each other by partitions called *septa* (sing. *septum*). As mentioned, the heart is a twin pump: the right side (right atrium and right ventricle) handles venous blood, the left side (left atrium and left ventricle) arterial blood. The independent function of the two sides of the heart is often acknowledged by referring to them as the "right heart" and the "left heart." The respective locations of the

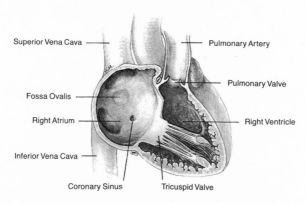

Figure 3. Right side of the heart shown with the front wall removed.

four chambers, as they appear when looking at the front surface of the heart, are shown in figure 2.

Venous blood enters the *right atrium* through two large veins and a small vein. The large veins, the *superior vena cava* and the *inferior vena cava,* channel blood from the upper and lower parts of the body, respectively. The third channel, the *coronary sinus,* delivers venous blood from the heart itself. The right atrium and its three tributary channels are shown in figure 3. The right atrium is an irregularly shaped chamber connecting, by way of a large opening, with the right ventricle. This orifice is protected by the *tricuspid valve.* The two large veins enter the atrium at its upper and lower right portions, respectively. The coronary sinus empties into the right atrium at its lower back wall. The mixture of blood derived from the three channels flows into the right ventricle through the tricuspid orifice. The right ventricle is divided into two portions: the lower portion, or inflow tract (behind the tricuspid valve); and the upper portion, or outflow tract, leading to the pulmonary orifice. At the top of the conical outflow tract is the pulmonary artery, separated from the tract by the outflow valve of the right side of the heart—the *pulmonary valve* (fig. 4). The contents of the right ventricle are ejected into the pulmonary artery, destined for the lungs.

The left side of the heart is almost identical in structure to the right side. The left atrium contains the orifices of four pulmonary veins, two of which drain blood from each lung. This atrium is

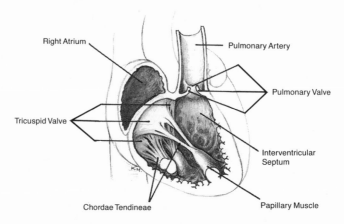

Figure 4. Details of the tricuspid and pulmonary valves.

located on the posterior (back) part of the heart; the pulmonary veins enter on its posterior surface. Its lower part is open, leading into the left ventricle. The connecting opening, the *mitral orifice,* contains the *mitral valve.* The left ventricle has a relatively small, conical cavity. The muscle of the left ventricle is three to four times thicker than that of the right ventricle. This relationship is in line with differences in pressure between the two sides of the heart. The upper part of the left ventricle contains both orifices: the inflow (mitral) orifice, to the left and rear, and the outflow (aortic) orifice, in front and to the right. The aorta originates from the left ventricle in a manner similar to that of the pulmonary artery from the right. Its origin contains the aortic valve (fig. 5).

As indicated, the two sides of the heart are separated from each other by partitions, or septa: the *atrial septum,* and the *ventricular septum.* The former consists of a thin layer of muscle, with the exception of an oval area where muscle is missing. This feature, the *fossa ovalis* (fig. 3), is a remnant of a valve, present in the embryo, which protected an orifice between the two atria through which blood could flow from the right atrium into the left atrium before birth (see chap. 11). The ventricular septum consists of a thick muscle continuous with the "free" walls of the left ventricle. It is thinned out in only one small area, underneath the aortic valves, where no muscle is present (*membranous septum*). A common

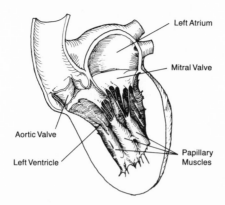

Figure 5. Details of the mitral and aortic valves.

birth defect is for this portion of the septum to be missing, providing a communication between the two ventricles.

The four heart valves consist of two sets almost identical in structure and function. The two inflow valves separate the atria from the
ventricles (*atrioventricular valves*). The two outflow valves separate the ventricles from the two main arterial trunks (*semilunar
valves*). The inflow valves prevent blood from backing into the atria
during ventricular contraction. The purpose of the semilunar
valves is to prevent the sucking back of blood from the aorta and
the pulmonary artery during ventricular relaxation.

The atrioventricular valves are attached to rings that form the
two orifices between atria and ventricles. These rings are made of
dense fibrous tissue (*annulus fibrosus*), and the valves themselves
are moderately thick, curtainlike structures. The right-sided atrioventricular valve, the tricuspid valve (fig. 4), has three leaflets; the
left-sided valve, the mitral valve, has two leaflets (fig. 5). Free
edges of each leaflet are connected through a series of delicate
strings or cords (*chordae tendineae*) with muscular outgrowths,
pillarlike structures, in the lower part of the ventricular cavity
(*papillary muscles*). Each ventricle has two such papillary muscles,
connected through the chordae tendineae with free edges of the
valve leaflets. These chordae fan out like a parachute to the edge of
the valve curtains. The papillary muscle and chordae tendineae
stabilize the valves and prevent their flapping back into the atrium
when they close in response to the high pressure in the ventricle.

The semilunar valves derive their name from their crescent-shaped leaflets. Each valve consists of three delicate leaflets, forced apart by high pressure during the ejection of blood into the aorta and the pulmonary artery. These leaflets, or cusps, stay close to the wall of the two arterial trunks, permitting free flow of blood. During the beginning of ventricular relaxation the cusps are sucked back with the blood and completely close the orifice separating the vessels from the ventricles during that portion of the heart cycle.

Structure of the Blood Vessels

The greater circulation consists of the aorta, the arteries, the arterioles, the capillary network, and the veins. The aorta, after arising from the left ventricle, sends off two coronary arteries and then runs upward (as the *ascending aorta*), arches to the left (*aortic arch*), and turns downward (descending aorta), in front of the spinal column, until it reaches the lower abdomen, where it divides into two principal branches. (The aorta and its more important branches are shown in figure 6.) The coronary arteries supply the heart itself; the aorta supplies blood to the head and upper extremities by means of four major arteries: two *carotid arteries* and two *subclavian arteries*. On the right side the carotid and subclavian originate as a joint, short trunk (*innominate artery*); on the left side they arise directly from the aorta. The aorta sends off no major branches until it passes below the diaphragm, where three major arteries originate from its frontal wall, and two from its side wall, supplying all abdominal organs. The branches of the *coeliac artery* supply the stomach, liver, spleen, and pancreas. The *renal artery* supplies the kidneys, and the *iliac artery* carries blood to the lower trunk and the legs. The *mesenteric artery* supplies the intestines.

The *coronary arteries* provide the blood supply for the heart itself (fig. 7). The *left coronary artery* runs a very short course and then divides into two large branches, the *anterior descending coronary artery* and the *left circumflex coronary artery*. The former supplies the front of the heart, particularly the left ventricle; the latter supplies the lower left portion, the back of the left ventricle, and the left atrium. The *right coronary artery* runs a moderately long course before dividing into branches; it supplies the right side of the heart and the lower back portion of the left ventricle. Even

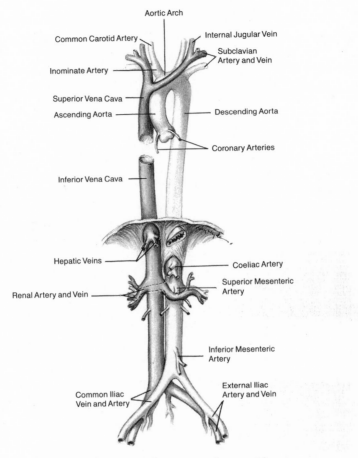

Figure 6. The principal arteries and veins. The heart has been removed from the illustration. Only initial portions of smaller vessels are shown.

though only two arteries originate from the aorta, the two branches of the left coronary artery are counted as major vessels; thus the clinician is used to thinking in terms of three, rather than two, sources of arterial blood supply to the heart.

The arteries in the body divide and subdivide into smaller segments. The smallest arterial branches, at the borderline of visibility, are called *arterioles,* beyond which the blood enters a myriad of

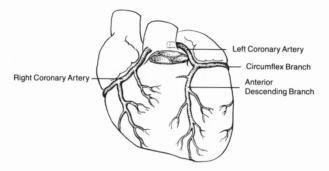

Figure 7. The coronary arterial circulation.

microscopic channels with very thin walls, the *capillaries*. These minute blood vessels are located within the tissues and organs of the body; they are integral parts of the various organ structures. The capillaries join together into very small veins, or *venules*, which in turn join together into increasingly large veins, eventually forming the two major veins, the superior and inferior vena cava. Larger veins usually accompany corresponding arteries and carry the same names, as indicated in figure 6. The inferior vena cava, the principal lower vein, is located alongside the aorta, deriving tributary veins similar to branches of the aorta. It drains blood from the abdomen and the lower part of the body into the right atrium. The large upper vein, the superior vena cava, drains blood from the head and upper extremities through four tributary veins analogous to the four corresponding arterial branches. It runs a short course in the chest, entering the upper portion of the right atrium.

The pulmonary circulation is presented in figure 8. Venous (dark) blood collected in the right atrium is pumped by the right ventricle into the pulmonary artery, which, after a short course upward, divides into two principal branches, each supplying one lung. The right and left branches of the pulmonary artery are large vessels, frequently referred to as the "right pulmonary artery" and "left pulmonary artery," in which case the pulmonary artery is called the "pulmonary trunk." Each artery divides into as many branches as there are lobes of the lungs (three on the right side and two on the left). These branches subdivide further into smaller and smaller branches, forming pulmonary arterioles and then pulmonary capillaries. The capillaries collect into venules and veins,

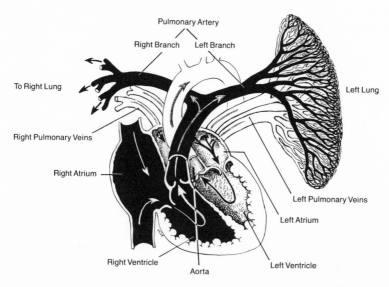

Figure 8. The pulmonary circulation. The right lung has been removed from the drawing. Oxygenated blood is shown in white and deoxygenated blood in black.

through which fully oxygenated blood returns to the left side of the heart. Four large veins, two from each lung, carry the blood to the left atrium.

The blood vessels show important structural differences, related to their various functions. The aorta and the largest of the arteries act as collectors and receptacles of blood; hence they are thick-walled and elastic. Smaller arteries participate in regulating blood flow and may require contraction and relaxation under certain conditions; hence their tissues are less elastic and more muscular. The arterioles have a particularly well-developed musculature; its contraction and relaxation is the principal factor in regulating blood pressure, as will be discussed later (chap. 3). The walls of the pulmonary artery are thinner than those of the aorta, as it is exposed to considerably lower pressure. Smaller pulmonary arteries and arterioles have poorly developed musculature, although in certain diseases this muscular tissue develops. The veins of the systemic and the pulmonary circuits are thin-walled, collapsible vessels in which blood flows under low pressure. Larger systemic veins have valves (similar to the semilunar valves of the heart) that prevent backflow of blood, particularly in parts of the body where blood flows against gravity.

The *lymphatic system* is an auxiliary system of blood vessels carrying a white tissue fluid (*lymph*) resembling blood plasma that participates in the nutritional process of organs. Most tissues of the body contain lymphatic capillaries, which collect certain elements of tissue fluid and carry it through a fine network into larger vessels and then into a large duct (*thoracic duct*) that runs upward along the thoracic spine and empties itself into a tributary of the superior vena cava. The lymph thus mixes with blood and becomes part of the blood plasma. Smaller lymphatic vessels are connected with lymph nodes, which act as important filters, extracting undesirable components of tissue fluid and preventing them from entering the bloodstream.

Chapter Two

The Normal Heart: Function

Cardiac Impulses and Their Conduction

The heart has the unique property of rhythmicity. To maintain life, it must contract rhythmically; the average rate of contraction of the heart for an adult at rest is seventy times a minute. Proper function of the circulatory system also requires a well-coordinated contraction of the various parts of the heart. The origin of the cardiac impulses and their conduction are the functions of specialized cells distributed throughout the heart, consisting of the *pacemaker* (the initiator of cardiac action) and the *conducting system* (the distributor of the impulses through the heart). These cells are grouped together into three types of structures: two larger accumulations of cells, or *nodes;* nervelike conduits, or *bundles,* with branches; and the terminal portion of the branches, constituting a fine network on the inner surface of the ventricles.

The uppermost node, the *sinoatrial node (S-A node),* is located at the junction of the superior vena cava and the right atrium. The lower node, the *atrioventricular node (A-V node),* is located in the lower septal wall of the right atrium. From the lower portion of the A-V node emerges the *bundle of His,* entering the junction between the two atria and the two ventricles, where it divides into two principal branches: the left-bundle branch and the right-bundle branch, which run down either side of the ventricular septum. The branches subdivide into smaller and smaller branches, eventually forming the fine network, or *Purkinje network,* located

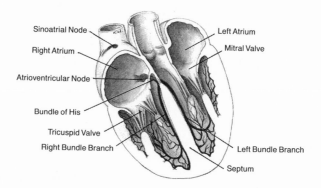

Figure 9. The heart with its front wall removed, shown to indicate the principal parts of the conduction system.

in the endocardial layer of the ventricles, where it comes in contact with muscle cells to be stimulated. A diagram of the conducting system is shown in figure 9.

Specialized cells of the S-A node generate electrical potential. When that potential reaches a certain level, it is discharged, activating the conducting system through which an electrical impulse travels, producing contraction of the cardiac muscle. The discharge of electrical potential in specialized cells is called *depolarization*. Immediately after depolarization the cell begins rebuilding electrical potential (*repolarization*) for the next impulse. This process is analogous to discharging and recharging a battery. All specialized cells have the capacity of generating an electrical impulse as well as carrying it rapidly throughout the conducting system. However, impulse formation in cells other than those of the S-A node is suppressed by the function of the S-A node, which as the *primary pacemaker* has the fastest rate of discharge. Its impulse directly stimulates the atria to contract, then speeds through the atrium to the A-V node, where it slows considerably. When the impulse reaches the junction between the A-V node and the bundle of His, it passes quickly through the remainder of the conducting system down to the Purkinje system, through which it stimulates the ventricles to contract. Slow conduction through the A-V node is essential for appropriate coordination of atrial and ventricular contractions, which should be separated by an interval of about 0.16 seconds to facilitate flow of blood from the atria to the ventricles.

Since all cells within the conducting system are capable of impulse formation, they serve as standby pacemakers activated only when the primary pacemaker fails to discharge. The lower portion of the A-V node, at its junction with the bundle of His, is the *secondary pacemaker.* Its rate of discharge, 50 times a minute, is slower than that of the primary pacemaker. Lower divisions of the conducting system, including the Purkinje network, represent the third line of defense against failure of the impulse to reach the ventricles. The discharge rate of this *tertiary pacemaker* is 30 to 40 times a minute. It is most frequently activated when the connection between the A-V node and the Purkinje system is interrupted, in which case the atria may contract at a fast rate, obeying the primary pacemaker, while the ventricles contract more slowly, activated by the tertiary pacemaker (see chap. 6).

The heart muscle, like other muscle tissue, has the ability to contract (that is, reduce its length), thereby exerting a considerable force. Since the heart muscle is globular in shape and envelopes a cavity filled with blood, its contraction expels most of the contents of the cavity. Muscle cells, accepting the stimulus from the conducting system, also discharge electrical potential while contracting (being depolarized) and are recharged (repolarized) during relaxation. However, these cells under normal conditions are not capable of impulse formation.

The primary pacemaker, the S-A node, is under the control of the autonomic nervous system (the part of the nervous system unresponsive to a person's will) through fibers connecting it with both divisions of the autonomic nervous system: sympathetic nerve fibers can quicken impulse formation; parasympathetic nerve fibers can slow it. This nervous control permits necessary adjustments in cardiac function, such as accelerating the heart rate during exercise and slowing it afterward. The secondary pacemaker is less efficiently regulated by the autonomic nervous system. The tertiary pacemaker has no significant connections with that system: its rate of discharge remains the same under all conditions.

Ejection of Blood

The pumping action of the heart results primarily from ventricular contraction. The atria act more as collecting reservoirs, and their

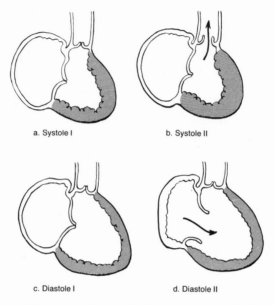

a. Systole I b. Systole II

c. Diastole I d. Diastole II

Figure 10. A ventricle during two stages of systole and two stages of diastole.

contraction accounts for only a small part of the blood entering the ventricles from the atria; most of it is sucked in by the ventricles. Since the state of contraction or relaxation of the ventricles determines the overall volume of the heart, it is customary to divide the cardiac cycle into two periods: the period of ventricular contraction, or *systole;* and the period of ventricular relaxation, or *diastole.*

During systole the beginning of ventricular contraction and the resulting first rise in the pressure inside the two ventricular chambers causes the two atrioventricular valves to close (fig. 10a). The sudden tensing of the atrioventricular valves produces a loud noise—the first heart sound. Now the pressure can effectively build within the ventricles as they contract, until it exceeds the pressure in the aorta and the pulmonary artery, at which point the two semilunar valves are forced open and blood begins to flow into the two arterial trunks (fig. 10b). Blood is pumped with considerable force and velocity during the first half of the ejection, and then gradually slows down. At the moment ventricular contraction ends and the period of relaxation begins (diastole), pressure in the cavities starts to fall, causing the semilunar valves to be sucked into closed position (fig. 10c). Closure of the semilunar valves produces the second heart sound. Relaxation of the ventricular muscle now produces a rapid fall in pressure in the two ventricular cavities, and the moment ventricular pressures fall below atrial pressures the two atrioventricular valves open widely, permitting the ventricle to fill with blood from the atria (fig. 10d). As stated, relaxation enlarges the ventricular cavities and sucks in atrial blood; this occurs mostly during the first third of the diastole; during the middle third relatively little pressure change and flow occur. This is the period of rest, *diastasis*. The final third of the diastole involves the contraction of the atria, at which time the small remainder of blood (20 percent of the total volume or less) enters the ventricle from the atria. From the above description two points are clear: (1) During both systole and diastole there are short periods of time during which flow of blood ceases; these occur between the time one set of valves closes and the other opens, as shown in figures 10a and 10c. These two periods are referred to as *isometric* contraction and relaxation of the cardiac muscle; they are important in permitting efficient and rapid rise and fall in pressure. (2) Flow through the two sets of orifices does not occur with uniform volume and velocity; maximum flow occurs during the earliest part of ventricular ejection and ventricular filling.

Blood Pressure and Blood Flow

During systole the semilunar valves are wide open, and the pressure within the cavities of the two ventricles and the arterial trunks on the respective sides is identical. The highest level of pressure within the ventricle and the arterial system on the corresponding side is called *systolic pressure*. The systolic pressure within the left ventricle and the aorta is about five times higher than the corresponding pressure within the right ventricle and the pulmonary artery. The onset of diastole and the closure of the semilunar valves signal the separation of pressure between the ventricles and the arterial trunks; pressures in the ventricular cavities drop sharply to levels close to zero; pressures in the aorta and pulmonary artery level off to a point slightly lower than that of semilunar-valve closure. The lowest pressure in the ventricles and the lowest pressure levels in the arterial trunks are termed *diastolic pressure*. Since during most of diastole pressures in the two ventricles and their respective atria are identical, ventricular diastolic pressure and atrial pressure are usually the same. Normal average pressures in the adult are as follows:

1. Systolic pressure in the arterial side of the systemic circulation (identical with systolic pressure in the left ventricle): 120 mm Hg
2. Diastolic pressure in the aorta and the systemic arteries: 80 mm Hg
3. Systolic pressure in the arterial side of the pulmonary circulation and in the right ventricle: 25 mm Hg
4. Diastolic pressure in the pulmonary artery and branches: 10 mm Hg
5. Pressure in the pulmonary venous side of the circulation, the left atrium, and the left ventricle during diastole: 8 mm Hg
6. Pressure in the systemic veins, the right atrium, and the right ventricle during diastole: 3 mm Hg

The heart, being a pressure pump, functions properly if it can maintain an adequate flow of blood and adequate pressure. Both blood flow and blood pressure have to be regulated in response to needs of the body. The quantity of blood ejected into each circulatory system—the volume of blood flow—is the *cardiac output.* Cardiac output can be expressed in two ways: either as the quantity of blood ejected into the arterial system with each ventricular contraction (*stroke volume*), expressed in cubic centimeters per heartbeat; or the total quantity of blood ejected into each arterial system within a minute (*minute volume*), expressed in liters per minute. It is customary to use the general term "cardiac output" to indicate minute volume and to specify stroke volume as such. The maintenance and regulation of cardiac output is one of the most intricate functions of the circulatory system; it will be discussed later in this chapter in connection with the physiology of exercise.

Blood pressure commonly refers to pressures in the systemic arterial circulation. The arterial blood pressure can be maintained at its level of 100 mm Hg or above only because the blood is enclosed within a system of vessels so regulated that the same amount of blood

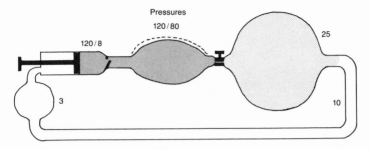

Figure 11. A circulatory model resembling the human circulation.

is pumped into it and discharged from it simultaneously. Thus if a stroke volume of 70 cc of blood is ejected into the aorta with each beat, an equal amount leaves the arterial system through the "exit"—the arterioles—into the capillary system. The arterial system is protected at one end by the aortic valves and at the other end by the sum total of the arterioles. A simplified diagram of such a system is provided in figure 11, in which a pump (at left) ejects fluid into an elastic container that has at its end a stopcock; that container is connected to a much larger container from which a system of tubes returns the fluid into the pump. The pump represents the left side of the heart; the first "closed" container, the high-pressure arterial system; the stopcock, the arterioles; the larger, "open" container, the capillary and venous reservoir of blood; the returning pipes, the larger veins; and the container at the lower left, the right atrium. The arterioles are normally in a semiconstricted state and are regulated by impulses reaching them from the central nervous system via the nerves. These impulses are capable of either constricting the arterioles further or relaxing them, thereby regulating outflow from the first reservoir and hence the arterial pressure. In the arterial system resistance to blood flow is very high; in the pulmonary arterial system, where arterioles are wide open, resistance and pressures are much lower than on the systemic side. The capillary and venous systems in both circuits have no narrow area offering any resistance to flow and hence their pressure is close to zero.

This relationship between pressure, flow, and resistance is usually presented in the form of an equation derivative of Poiseuille's law and analogous to Ohm's law in electricity: *pressure* equals *flow* (cardiac output) times *resistance*, or $P = F \times R$. It follows that pressure can be maintained at a constant level only if resistance falls each time cardiac output increases. This actually takes place because of a barostat, a mechanism analogous to the thermostat that regulates pressure rather than temperature. The human barostat consists of pressure-sensitive points within the walls of some arteries. If the volume of blood ejected into the aorta increases, raising the cardiac output, the aorta becomes distended. Pressure-sensitive receptors react to the distension of arterial walls by sending signals through the nervous system to relax the arterioles just enough to let the excess blood out of the arterial system and to maintain constant arterial pressure.

The systemic circulation consists of many circuits connected in parallel (see fig. 1, p. 2). Each of these smaller circuits has its own resistance at the arteriolar level. The general equation mentioned above applies to each of these circuits as well as to their sum total; consequently, arteriolar resistance in each region determines blood flow independently within the systemic flow and pressure available. Thus, if in a given organ the arterioles were to constrict, its blood supply would be reduced, since blood would flow more easily through alternate circuits; if the arterioles relaxed in a given circuit, blood flow would increase proportionally. This mechanism, mediated less through the central nervous system than through local reflexes, controls blood flow through individual organs and parts of the body. Such a regulating mechanism (*regional flow control*) provides for increased blood flow in areas where it is most needed. Thus during exercise the working muscles receive a more abundant blood supply, and after meals the digestive tract is provided with increased blood flow—all without disrupting the general balance of the total flow or altering the arterial pressure in the systemic circulation.

The blood pressure is the same in all arteries up to the beginning of the arterioles. There the pressure falls abruptly from a systolic level of 120 mm Hg to 25 mm Hg in the capillaries, a level just sufficient to drive the blood into the venous system through the narrow capillary channels. On the venous side blood flows slowly toward the heart. The veins have virtually no driving power, and the blood flow is aided only by the venous valves and by the massaging action of the various muscles of the body.

The aorta and its principal branches are, as mentioned, elastic vessels. This property plays an important part in causing the blood to flow through the body evenly rather than intermittently. During systole all the elastic arteries are expanded by the addition of blood ejected from the left ventricle; the elastic vessels then revert to their original size as the excess blood drains into the capillaries. If blood were ejected into a system of totally rigid pipes, then forward flow of blood would occur only during systole and would stop during diastole. Elastic tissue in arterial walls makes for a reservoir of variable capacity that acts as a pressure and flow equalizer. This principle is often used in perfume and cologne atomizers: simple dispensers with one bulb spray only when the bulb is squeezed; dispensers with a double bulb are capable of spraying continuously because the second bulb, which is not squeezed, distends with air when the first bulb is squeezed and acts as a pressure and flow equalizer.

The sudden dilation of the aorta by the blood ejected from the left ventricle is transmitted along the arterial system as a wave of elastic displacement of the arterial wall, usually referred to as the *arterial pulse*. The pulse is an index of the heart rate but also reflects the quantity of blood ejected into the aorta, the mode of its injection, the elasticity of the larger arteries, and the condition of the closed arterial system. It obviously provides important and readily obtainable information concerning the circulatory apparatus. Study of the arterial pulse has been a basis of diagnosing disease for many centuries.

The circulation through the pulmonary circuit is much simpler than the systemic circulation. It is confined to a single organ, the lungs; therefore there is little need for the regulation of blood flow (see fig. 1). Its pressure is low because, under normal circumstances, pulmonary arterioles are wide open and offer little resistance to flow, and nervous regulation of pulmonary arterioles is practically nonexistent. Consequently, the fall in pressure from the arteriolar side to the capillary side of the pulmonary circulation (*pressure gradient*) is very low, less than 10 mm Hg.

The final destination of the circulatory system is the capillary network in both circuits. In it the exchange between blood and tissue, and between blood and air, takes place. The thin walls of the capillaries are a semipermeable membrane, a partition through which certain chemical substances can pass back and forth: gases, water, and simple chemical substances, such as sodium, potassium, and glucose can leave or enter the blood as needed, but blood cells and large molecules (for example, proteins) remain in the blood. The capillaries thus act as an intermediary in two vital body functions: (1) blood-gas exchange, the acquisition of oxygen in the lungs and its delivery to the tissues coupled with the taking of carbon dioxide from the tissues and its excretion through the lungs (by means of a chemical reaction between the gases and hemoglobin, the red dye contained in the red blood cells); and (2) the physical process of regulating the water content in the tissues and blood and permitting an exchange of electrolytes (such as sodium and potassium) between tissue fluid and the blood. Water and chemical substances dissolved in the blood plasma can enter and exit as needed, driven by two forces: the osmotic pressure on the two sides of the capillary walls and the hydrostatic pressure within them. Each substance dissolved in the blood on one side of the capillary wall, and in the tissue fluid on its other side, reaches equal concentration in the two media. The pressure in the capillaries, about 25 mm Hg, maintains a fluid balance within the vascular system, as this pressure is identical with the osmotic pressure exerted by plasma proteins and electrolytes. If the hydrostatic pressure increases, or the osmotic pressure falls, then fluid leaves the vascular system, increasing the fluid content of tissues—a situation that may lead to edema (see chap. 5). A fall in hydrostatic pressure or increase in osmotic pressure draws fluid into the vascular system, raising the volume of circulating blood. These factors play an important role in maintaining blood volume at an optimal level. Water and solutes are quickly and efficiently exchanged in the capillary system.

Exercise

The circulatory system supplies oxygen and other vital substances to tissues of the body. Obviously, the demands on this supply line increase sharply during exercise. Human energy is customarily expressed in terms of *oxygen consumption;* oxygen consumption is to the body what gasoline consumption is to the automobile. Oxygen consumption is at its minimum during complete rest (*resting oxygen consumption*) and measures in an average adult between

200 and 250 cc of oxygen per minute. This level (1 MET) covers the essential metabolic needs of the body (*basal metabolism*). The level of oxygen consumption rises steeply with activity since the oxygen cost of human effort is quite high. For example, walking at a moderate pace increases oxygen consumption to about three times its basal level. Strenuous exercise, such as climbing stairs briskly or running, may increase the basal demands for oxygen by as much as five to eight times. Maximum possible effort for a healthy individual occurs at the cost of 10 to 15 times the basal oxygen consumption; for a trained athlete it may reach 20 times the resting level. This high need for oxygen is one of the principal limiting factors of human exercise. The limitation depends on the possible top performance of the two principal systems involved in the process: respiration, supplying enough oxygen to the air spaces of the lungs; and circulation, delivering enough oxygen to the working tissues.

The burden of delivering 10 to 20 times the basal amount of oxygen to the tissues is considerable, and it is supportable only because of work-saving adaptive mechanisms. These mechanisms apply primarily to the circulatory apparatus, since the respiration is usually capable of increasing its work in proportion to high demands. The circulatory system is so designed that delivery of oxygen can increase much more than the work of the heart and circulation can. This is made possible through three adaptive mechanisms. First, in periods of high demand the circulatory system makes full use of the available oxygen supply. Normally during rest only a small part of the available oxygen is consumed by the tissues. Blood returning to the right side of the heart is, at rest, still 75 percent saturated with oxygen, indicating that only one-fourth of the available supply has been utilized. Better utilization of oxygen is an effective work-saving device for the heart. For example, if a certain form of exercise demands four times the resting amount of oxygen, the tissue can easily draw twice as much oxygen as during rest (reducing the oxygen saturation of the returning venous blood from 75 percent to 50 percent), in which case the volume of blood circulating through the tissues (cardiac output) has only to double instead of quadruple to meet the full demand. Second, blood can be redistributed (by way of regional flow regulation, as discussed earlier) so that the working muscles or organs get a greater share of the flow than do less important regions. Thus during exercise the digestive tract, the kidneys, the brain, the skin, and other nonparticipating organs are perfused with less blood than during rest in order to supply the heart and the working muscles with more oxygen. Third, working muscles can perform temporarily with a smaller supply of oxygen than needed to meet actual energy demands. This "oxygen debt" is repaid immediately after exercise ceases. This mechanism is particularly important for short-term, high-intensity forms of exercise.

These adaptive mechanisms are essential, since the heart has a rather limited capacity for increasing its work. It is estimated that in a healthy individual, cardiac output can only increase to four or at most five times its resting level (from a normal of 5 liters per minute to 20 or 25 liters per minute). Thus, as a general rule, at peak cardiac performance the potential oxygen supply to the tissues rises fourfold; the tissues can extract up to four times as much oxygen from the blood during exercise than at rest; therefore top muscular performance is about 16 times the resting level when expressed in terms of oxygen consumption.

The following analogy may help illustrate the adaptive circulatory process during exercise. Let us imagine a large industrial plant with ample supplies of raw material but no storage facilities for its principal fuel, coal, which has to be brought in. The normal daily manufacturing activities of the plant require a quantity of coal equivalent to five carloads; however, since the shortest train consists of 20 cars, only one-quarter of each car is unloaded, thereby supplying the needs. At times the plant is called on to increase temporarily the manufacture of one of its principal products. The increased fuel demands are met in part by bringing in longer trains, and in part by unloading more coal from each car. The plant can also, to conserve fuel, slow down or eliminate the manufacture of some less essential product. If one assumes that the rail-loading facilities at the other end of the communication line limit coal delivery to 80 carloads a day, the maximum manufacturing capabilities of the plant would amount to 16 times its ordinary level, if all 80 carloads were brought in and all the coal in them unloaded.

Physiologists and clinicians often find it necessary to calculate the work of the heart, at rest and during exercise, in terms of work delivered (*external work*) rather than the actual energy utilized by the heart. External work is expressed by the following formula: *work* equals *blood pressure* times *cardiac output*, or

$W = P \times F$. The increase in work during exercise is directly related to the increase in cardiac output, since blood pressure shows little change, its level being well regulated by the previously described barostatic mechanism.

In spite of the efficient work-saving devices for the heart and the circulation operating in the healthy individual, exercise imposes a heavy strain on the circulatory system. Obviously, under conditions of less than perfect health, certain functions of the circulation begin to lag, and the efficiency of the circulatory adjustment may suffer. Exercise, which may reveal faulty circulatory function long before it becomes evident under resting conditions, thus provides one of the fundamental tests of the circulatory apparatus in the study of cardiac disease.

Chapter Three

Diagnosis

Case Finding

The discovery of a previously unknown health problem, or case finding, may occur when an abnormality is found during the routine medical examination of a healthy patient or when a person becomes aware of a change in his or her state of health and seeks medical care. Periodic health examinations and examinations requested by someone's employer or insurer vary greatly in scope and thoroughness. A physical examination is mandatory. A variety of tests may be included in the examination, such as blood tests, an electrocardiogram, a chest X-ray, and treadmill stress tests. Some findings raise suspicion that a heart problem may be present:

abnormal heart sounds or murmurs

irregularities of the rhythm of the heart

elevated blood pressure

unusual shape or enlargement of the heart shadow in the X-ray film

abnormalities shown in the standard electrocardiogram

electrocardiographic abnormalities detected during a treadmill
    stress test

The discovery of an abnormality in a routine examination usually results in further evaluation to confirm or reject the suspicion of heart disease. Occasionally, findings are characteristic enough to make a firm diagnosis at once. Heart disease present at birth—congenital heart disease—may be discovered in the postnatal examination or in a periodic examination performed during the first year of life.

The discovery of a previously unknown heart abnormality is a goal of preventive cardiology, but the commonest way heart disease is first detected is when a person becomes aware of certain symptoms and seeks medical care. Symptoms may signal an acute change in the state of health, requiring immediate attention, or they may be nondisabling and repetitive.

Acute events that may demand emergency medical care include sudden loss of consciousness, severe dizziness or faintness, severe chest pain, severe shortness of breath, or sudden onset of rapid heart action. Chronic or repetitive symptoms that most frequently lead to the discovery of heart disease are shortness of breath, chest pain, and palpitations.

Shortness of breath is a normal response to strenuous exercise and as such is not alarming. However, shortness of breath provoked by minor, previously well-tolerated activity or occurring during rest makes a patient aware of an abnormal respiratory effort. This abnormal shortness of breath, most often associated with diseases of the heart or lungs, is called *dyspnea*. Dyspnea may appear in patients resting in bed as a sudden onset of rapid breathing, often accompanied by coughing, or as discomfort when lying down if the patient can breathe comfortably only when sitting up. A special variety of dyspnea, hyperventilation, in which a person is compelled to breathe deeply and rapidly, is usually unrelated to serious abnormalities of the heart, being a response to abnormal signals from the brain that may occur in some anxious, otherwise healthy persons. As a manifestation of heart disease, dyspnea is usually related to impaired function of the left ventricle (see chap. 5).

Chest pain is the principal symptom of coronary disease. Inasmuch as chest pain may be produced by a variety of conditions, some inconsequential, identification of the cause of chest pain constitutes a real challenge to the physician. Other causes of chest pain include pericarditis, aortic dissection, spasm of the esophagus, and pleurisy. In many cases, chest pain originates in the muscles or nerves within the chest wall and does not indicate a significant health problem.

Ordinarily a person is not aware of the beating of the heart, although it often seems to "pound" during strenuous exercise, excitement, or fright. Palpitations refer to unprovoked perception of unusual heart action, often occurring at rest. A patient may recognize the heart beating too slowly, too fast, or irregularly. Thus palpitations suggest an abnormality of the rhythm of the heart (*arrhythmia*).

These three symptoms motivating a person to seek medical care account for the majority of discoveries of a previously unknown heart disease. They may, however, indicate a health problem of a different nature, or none at all. Less frequently, heart disease is discovered in patients who consult physicians for other symptoms: dizziness, excessive weakness, fainting attacks, swelling of ankles, abdominal discomfort, and so on.

The Initial Medical Examination

In the initial contact with a patient suspected of having heart disease, the physician takes a complete medical history and performs a physical examination. The medical history is largely devoted to a detailed analysis of the patient's symptoms. The patient's ability to present a well-observed, reliable, and consistent account of symptoms is essential in helping the physician draw correct conclusions. The medical history also includes background information, such as past medical problems, a family medical history, a social and occupational assessment, and an evaluation of the patient's personality.

During the initial interview the physician takes note of the patient's general appearance and his or her concern regarding the possibility of serious illness. Certain abnormalities may become obvious: shortness of breath while talking, unusual pallor, cyanosis, and strain in performing minor activities such as walking into the room or dressing. Such observations do not necessarily point to a heart problem but could, supported by the patient's history, make the physician suspect heart disease.

A complete physical examination focuses on those areas of concern revealed in the history taking and initial observations. The contribution of the physical examination to the diagnosis of heart disease varies widely: sometimes, although serious heart disease is present, the findings of the physical examination may be normal; at other times, a definitive diagnosis can be made on the basis of the medical history and physical examination without further tests.

Cardiac auscultation—listening to the heart with a stethoscope on the front of the chest—is an important part of the examination. In a healthy person cardiac auscultation reveals two normal heart sounds produced by the action of heart valves. Abnormal findings suggesting heart disease include certain alterations of the normal sounds and the presence of additional sounds and heart murmurs. Heart murmurs occur when a normal, smooth, "laminar" blood flow becomes turbulent. Turbulence arises when there is an obstacle in the path of blood flow, such as narrowing of a heart valve, backflow through an incompetent heart valve, or an abnormal communication between the right and the left sides of the heart or between certain large blood vessels. (Murmur due to turbulent flow may be present in healthy subjects as well, particularly in children after acceleration or increase of blood flow such as during exercise. Such murmurs are usually referred to as "functional" or "innocent.") Thus the discovery of a heart murmur can help the physician diagnose diseases of heart valves and certain congenital defects of the heart. Other abnormal findings on auscultation include a "friction rub," usually indicating pericarditis; extra heart sounds, which may be related to impaired function of the heart; and abnormal clicks or snaps originating in malfunctioning valves.

Other parts of the physical examination providing diagnostic information in heart disease include taking the arterial pulse, observing the venous pulse, and measuring the blood pressure. Serious malfunction of the heart (*congestive heart failure*) may be signaled by abnormalities of the venous pulse in the neck, the presence of rales (bubbling noises during breathing), enlargement of the liver, and the accumulation of fluid in the ankles, around the lungs, and in the abdominal cavity. A physician can perceive abnormalities of the heart rhythm by feeling the pulse at the wrist. However, a more detailed analysis requires listening to the sequence of heartbeats with the stethoscope, sometimes combined with observing the venous pulse.

After completing the medical history and physical examination, the physician can sometimes establish a definitive diagnosis or rule out heart disease. Usually, however, the result of the initial workup is a tentative diagnosis or a list of illnesses to be considered. The next step is to select further diagnostic procedures. A wide range of tests is now available to aid in the diagnosis of heart disease, from simple ones performed in the office to complex hospital procedures, some entailing risk to the patient. It is customary to classify diagnostic heart tests as *noninvasive*, wherein all instruments used in the test remain outside the body, and *invasive*, requiring the introduction of catheters or other instruments into the body. Invasive diagnostic procedures also include certain minor operations.

Noninvasive Tests

Electrocardiography is one of the two oldest, most widely used, and least expensive tests in the diagnosis of heart disease. The *electrocardiogram*, developed for practical use at the turn of the century, records the electrical potential generated by each heartbeat. The contraction and relaxation of the heart muscle is caused by a flow of electrolytes (sodium, potassium, and calcium) in and out of each muscle cell through the surrounding membrane. This flow generates a weak electrical current. Each muscle cell of the heart is a miniature battery discharging electricity with each contraction (depolarizing), and recharging itself during relaxation (repolarizing). The electrocardiograph is an amplifier capable of picking up this weak current from the surface of the body. The electrical potential generated over time by the millions of heart muscle cells—between 0.1 and 2.0 millivolts, or about one millionth the voltage of household current—displayed continuously on a roll of graph paper, is the standard electrocardiogram. It consists of 12 leads recorded with electrodes placed on various points on the chest, both arms, and the left leg, thus providing electrical "views" of the heart from various angles.

An electrocardiographic image produced by a single heartbeat is shown in figure 12. Any deviation from the horizontal line, or *baseline*, whether above (*positive potential*) or below (*negative potential*), denotes electrical activity. Each change of potential is called a *wave*. The first is a positive, broad, triangular wave called the P *wave*, representing depolarization of the two atria and signaling their contraction. It is followed by a return to the baseline, called the *P-R interval*. Next comes a complex consisting of three sharp waves: a small, negative Q *wave*, a tall, positive R *wave*, and a small, negative S *wave*. These three waves together constitute the *QRS complex*, which shows depolarization of the two ventricles

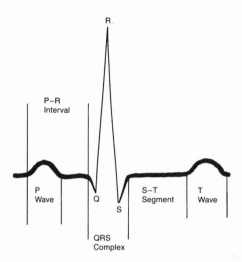

Figure 12. A typical electrocardiographic
lead showing the various components of
the electrocardiogram.

coinciding with the onset of ventricular contraction. A flat, electrically inert baseline follows (the *S-T segment*), after which the slower and lower *T wave* appears, indicating repolarization of the two ventricles. The section of the electrocardiogram including the QRS complex, the S-T segment, and the T wave is referred to as the *ventricular complex*. The end of the ventricular contraction occurs during the descending part of the T wave. Absence of electrical activity is displayed by the horizontal baseline between the end of the T wave and the beginning of the P wave of the next beat, during which time the ventricles relax.

The normal electrocardiogram shows a sequence of evenly spaced complexes. Experience has established the limits of normal variation in the height and direction of the five waves in healthy persons according to age group. The abnormal electrocardiogram may indicate two types of deviation from these norms: abnormalities of the sequence of beat (arrhythmias) and abnormalities of the waves and the baseline segments between them (abnormalities of electrocardiographic contour). The normal heart beats evenly at a rate ranging between 60 and 150 beats a minute. Irregular spacing of heartbeats demonstrates an arrhythmia, a disturbance of the rhythm of the heart. The electrocardiogram is the principal tool for diagnosing cardiac arrhythmias, since it shows the rate and regularity of heartbeats; the shape, direction, and relationship of the P waves to the other complexes, including the absence of P waves; and deviations in the contour of the QRS complexes and T waves in the abnormally spaced beats.

The electrocardiogram is an indispensable tool in recognizing and analyzing arrhythmias. An equally important role of the electrocardiogram is to provide information concerning the state of the heart muscle on the basis of certain alterations in the electrocardiographic complexes, especially the QRS-T part. This feature of the electrocardiogram, however, requires more cautious interpretation because alterations produced by changes in the heart muscle are less specific than those produced by arrhythmias. Alterations in the electrocardiogram helpful to the physician may result from myocardial infarction and from enlargement of one or both cardiac ventricles or atria. These changes tend to be a permanent feature of a given person's electrocardiogram. In addition, daily and hourly variations may suggest acute changes in the state of the heart muscle, such as ischemia, acute pericarditis, and imbalance of electrolytes. In some healthy persons electrocardiograms may deviate from the norm without indicating any heart problem; these are referred to as normal variants. By contrast, many electrocardiographic abnormalities—perhaps the majority—are inconclusive, or "nonspecific." Here the significance of the changes has to be evaluated by means other than the electrocardiogram.

Electrocardiography is the most universally and frequently used aid in the diagnosis of heart disease. Yet it has its limitations: a normal electrocardiogram can be present in patients with a serious heart problem, and an abnormal electrocardiogram does not automatically indicate significant heart disease.

Electrocardiographic techniques are also incorporated in certain other cardiac tests. The *treadmill stress test* helps evaluate the effect of increased work on the heart by monitoring it electrocardiographically while the patient exercises on a treadmill. The principal indication for this test is a suspicion of coronary-artery disease, which may reduce the oxygen supply to some part of the heart muscle (ischemia) during exercise. Occasionally exercise may provoke arrhythmias (see chap. 8), and this test is used to detect them. The *Holter monitor test* is a 24-hour survey of heart rhythm. The

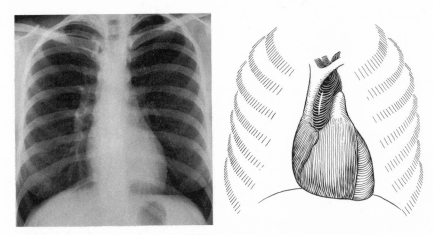

Figure 13. A radiograph (X-ray) of the chest in the anteroposterior view in a healthy person (left). A reference diagram (right) shows the heart and the great vessels in relation to the rib cage. Compare with figure 2 to identify cardiovascular structures.

patient wears a specialized tape recorder that registers every heartbeat. A computer analysis of the recording reveals any disturbances of heart rhythm. Newer, high-fidelity recording equipment may pick up indications of ischemia of the heart muscle. The electrocardiogram is an important aid in diagnosing some acute diseases of the heart or monitoring the heart during surgical procedures (cardiac or noncardiac). In such cases the heart rhythm is sensed by one or two electrocardiographic leads and is displayed continuously on an oscilloscope. This procedure is standard in intensive-care wards, including coronary-care units.

Radiography is the second traditional diagnostic aid in heart diseases. Because X rays penetrate certain tissues better than others, X-ray photography permits considerable differentiation of body structures. The chest X ray displays three types of shadows: the heavy shadow of bony structures (spine, ribs), the light shadow of lungs filled with air, and the intermediate shadow of the heart and blood vessels (fig. 13).

Radiographic examination can display enlargement of the heart and the great vessels arising from it as well as the distribution of blood vessels throughout the lungs. Newer technology (especially echocardiography) provides a more accurate method of recognizing enlargement of the individual heart chambers or other structures in the X-ray shadow of the heart. Today cardiac radiography is used more as a screening technique and a means of assessing changes occurring between examinations than as a way of definitively diagnosing cardiac enlargment. This test, however, is indispensable in displaying fluid in the lungs, an important feature of heart failure. (Current technology has produced some specialized radiological techniques in diagnosing heart disease. These will be discussed later in the chapter in connection with invasive tests.)

Blood tests usually play an important role in diagnosing diseases, but not in the case of heart ailments. Only three sets of blood tests are a regular part of diagnostic work in cardiology: measurement of cardiac enzymes in acute myocardial infarction; measurement of cardiac drug levels in the blood to regulate dosage; and blood culture for discovery of bacteria if infection of the heart is suspected.

Echocardiography has revolutionized the diagnosis of heart disease since it was first applied in the 1960s. Like other ultrasound techniques, it produces an image by transmitting high-frequency sound waves (ultrasound), which reflect off different structures of the body with varying intensity; the resulting data show the interface of those structures.

In the original echocardiographic technique, an electronic wand—a transducer—is pressed against the patient's chest and pointed in the direction of the heart, toward which it sends ultrasonic waves. The heart muscle, its neighboring structures, and cavities filled with blood vary in density, and the transducer picks up those variations in the reflected sound, which it converts into an electronic signal that is recorded on moving paper. The echocardiographic record shows not only changes in the size of the cardiac chambers during ventricular contraction and relaxation but also the rapidity of contraction and relaxation—points of some importance in evaluating heart function. This method, *M-mode echocardiography*, displays a one-dimensional view of the portion of the heart at which the transducer is aimed. It is often referred to as the "icepick" view of the heart because the narrow sound beam drives straight through the heart like an icepick through a solid block (fig. 14). M-mode echocardiographic display provides some information that previously required invasive tests, such as the size (width) of each heart chamber, the thickness of the mus-

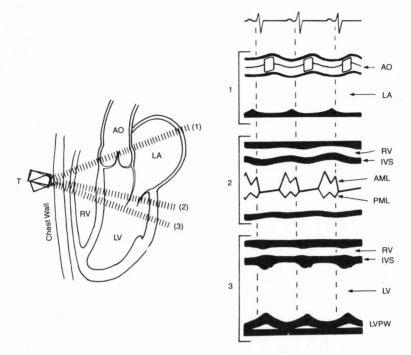

Figure 14. A normal M-mode (unidimensional) echocardiographic image. The left side of the diagram presents three standard directions of the ultrasonic beam, with cardiac structures identified. The right side shows a record of the echocardiographic images in each position as recorded on moving paper. Abbreviations: AO, aorta; LA, left atrium; RV, right ventricle; LV, left ventricle; IVS, interventricular septum; AML, anterior leaflet of the mitral valves; PML, posterior leaflet of the mitral valves; LVPW, posterior wall of the left ventricle. (Reprinted, by permission, from Arthur Selzer, *Principles and Practice of Clinical Cardiology* [Philadelphia: W. B. Saunders, 1983].)

cle of the ventricle, change in the size of the left ventricle between systole and diastole (the rate of change reflects its efficiency), the presence of fluid between the two layers of the pericardium, and the presence of abnormal structures (clots, tumors) within the cavities of the heart.

In the late 1970s a new technology was developed in the field of echocardiography permitting two-dimensional imaging. Instead of sending a single ultrasonic beam, the transducer now sends an oscillating series of beams along a single plane shaped like a large

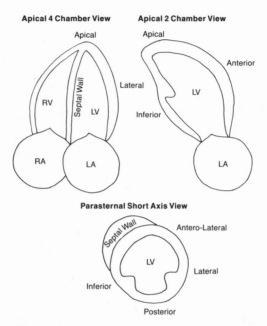

Figure 15. The three standard views of two-dimensional echocardiographic images. The various structures are identified, including five segments of the left ventricular walls. The images are recorded on a videotape, which permits viewing cardiac structure in real-time motion. Abbreviations: LV, left ventricle; LA, left atrium; RV, right ventricle; RA, right atrium. (Reprinted, by permission, from Arthur Selzer, *Principles and Practice of Clinical Cardiology* [Philadelphia: W. B. Saunders, 1983].)

slice of pie (60° to 90° of a circle). The information obtained from these echoes is processed by computer, then displayed on an oscilloscope and recorded on videotape. This technique has widened the application of echocardiography by displaying details of the interior of the heart and its various parts in motion in real time (fig. 15). It allows the cardiologist to detect abnormalities in the size, shape, and mode of contraction of each cardiac chamber, in the contraction of specific portions of the ventricular muscle, and in the thickness of cardiac valves and the size of their opening. It also can reveal clots, vegetations, or tumors inside the heart and aid in the diagnosis of certain congenital abnormalities of the heart.

Further technological advances have applied the Doppler effect to echocardiography as a means of studying blood flow through the heart. This physical principle describes the effect of motion on sound waves: a person listening to a sound will perceive a rise in pitch if the source of the sound is approaching and a fall in pitch if the source is receding. In echocardiography the Doppler effect lets us measure the velocity of blood flow toward or away from the transducer. On the videotape these changes in velocity and direction of blood flow are displayed as variations in color. *Doppler echocardiography* can show the presence and approximate volume of backflow through incompetent heart valves. It also aids in evaluating shunts through abnormal communications within the heart in some types of congenital heart disease and in gauging the severity of stenosis (narrowing) of a cardiac valve as well as approximate pressures in certain parts of the heart and great vessels. Doppler echocardiography has introduced an entirely new approach to noninvasive diagnosis: whereas conventional echocardiography opened up the field of noninvasive diagnosis of structural abnormalities of the heart, Doppler echocardiography has made it possible to evaluate the dynamics of blood flow through the heart.

Another echocardiographic technique is *transesophageal echocardiography,* in which the transducer is placed at the end of a tube similar to that used in endoscopic examination of the stomach and esophagus. This tube is swallowed by the patient, and the transducer is lowered to the level of the heart. Since the esophagus lies immediately behind the heart, the beam does not have to pass through outer structures of the chest. Transesophageal echocardiography is thus capable of displaying images in much greater detail than conventional echocardiography. The procedure has its disadvantages, however; it cannot properly be considered noninvasive, and it causes the patient some discomfort. This technique is sometimes used to monitor the heart and its responses during certain open-heart operations. Its value in diagnostic work has not yet been completely defined, but at present it is used to evaluate some special problems when conventional techniques are inconclusive.

Echocardiography has radically altered the approach to diagnosing heart disease. However, it is a very expensive test; hence it is used to evaluate specific problems and is not included in a routine examination. Many problems previously requiring complex invasive tests can now be adequately reviewed by echocardiography.

Other diagnostic tools involve injecting radioactive substances into the bloodstream. Such testing is the responsibility of a separate medical specialty, *nuclear medicine.* Although the field got its start in the 1920s, the primary application of nuclear techniques to heart disease was in research until the 1970s, when diagnostic tests were developed. Today nuclear cardiology is used extensively in diagnosis as well as research. Two important tests are *myocardial isotopic perfusion imaging,* in connection with exercise or pharmacological stress tests, and *nuclear ventriculography,* a method of studying the contraction and relaxation of the ventricles.

Perfusion tracer agents such as thallium-201 or Technetium 99_m Sestamibi are injected into the bloodstream and enter the heart muscle along with the coronary blood flow. The radioactivity disappears within a few days. Their presence in the heart muscle can be detected by a special camera. Thus, if a portion of the heart muscle is receiving less blood or is totally deprived of blood, it will show in the photographs as an area of lighter contrast or as a blank space.

The myocardial stress perfusion test discriminates between areas of the heart muscle permanently deprived of blood supply and those rendered temporarily ischemic (fig. 16). It is usually performed in connection with a treadmill test. Just before the end of the exercise, the liquid containing the thallium isotope is injected into the bloodstream. It may be performed by using a drug stress, such as diphridamole or adenosine, in patients who are unable to do a treadmill stress test. A symmetrical, full distribution of radioactive isotopes indicates good blood supply to the heart. If an area of abnormally reduced flow is found, another count is performed four hours later (occasionally a third count is taken 24 hours later). If the defect in the image remains unchanged, the physician can conclude that the area is permanently deprived of blood flow, probably a scar from a previous myocardial infarction. If, however, the abnormality has disappeared, the proper diagnosis is ischemia, temporary blockage of blood supply, usually owing to significant coronary-artery disease.

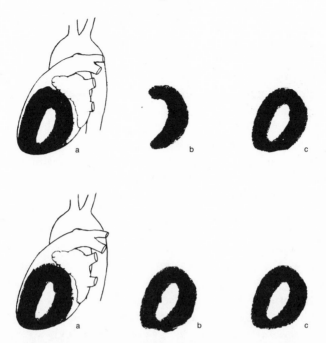

Figure 16. Thallium perfusion scintigram (image of thallium content of the heart used in thallium treadmill stress tests). The upper row shows a test positive for myocardial ischemia; the lower row shows results of such a test in a healthy person. (a) Lateral thallium image of the left ventricle superimposed on the heart. (b) Thallium images taken immediately after exercise. The upper drawing shows a large defect (absence of blood flow) of the anterior wall of the heart. The lower drawing shows normal perfusion. (c) Thallium images taken four hours after the exercise test, showing restoration of blood flow to a normal level. If the defect in the upper row present in b would persist in c, the test would be interpreted as showing a scar from past myocardial infarction rather than myocardial ischemia.

Nuclear ventriculography is a method of recording the motion of the heart chambers. The blood is made temporarily radioactive by injecting into the bloodstream an isotope with a very short half-life (a few hours). The isotope in the blood lining the cavities of the cardiac chambers permits observation, on videotape, of the heart in motion during the cardiac cycle. The function of each ventricle can be assessed from the extent of the motion of its walls. The test helps in calculating an important index of ventricular function, the *ejection fraction*, the ratio of the blood ejected during systole to the greatest volume of the ventricle in diastole. In addition, if the motion of the ventricular wall is abnormal, the test can reveal whether the entire ventricle is contracting sluggishly or only some parts of it. This wall motion abnormality is central to the diagnosis of coronary-artery disease.

The field of diagnostic imaging—cardiac imaging in particular—shows rapid advances. New isotopes are being developed in radiopharmacology that may refine the diagnostic value of present methods and introduce new tests. Most of the new techniques are first applied in research; only if their value in diagnosing individual cases of heart disease is demonstrated do they become generally available. The new technologies often require complex equipment costing millions of dollars. Two imaging techniques are widely used. *Computed axial tomography (CAT scan)* is an X-ray technique that allows the photographing of two-dimensional "slices" through parts of the body. The resulting image is assembled and enhanced by computer. At present, the CAT scan has little application in diagnosing abnormalities of the heart itself, but it is of value in addressing certain problems of the great vessels or the pericardium. *Magnetic resonance imaging* generates images of internal body structures by picking up changes in cells produced by exposure to a powerful magnet. This method, too, is limited in its application to cardiac diagnosis, though it may reveal tumors of the heart and abnormalities of the pericardium. Further developments in imaging are now being tested for research purposes, such as magnetic resonance spectroscopy and positron emission tomographic imaging, both of which may help in studying metabolic changes in the heart muscle and may lead to improvements in diagnosing special cardiac problems.

Invasive Tests

The heart is a pump that drives blood into the two great vessels and maintains adequate pressure to ensure proper blood supply throughout the body. The relationship of flow and pressure in the two circulations and their respective changes are called *hemodynamics*. At one time hemodynamic information could only be inferred from certain observations or extrapolated from animal measurements. A new era in cardiology arrived when hemodynamic measurements became possible in humans by means of *cardiac catheterization*. The technique of introducing a catheter, or thin tube, into the heart was demonstrated in Germany in 1929, but cardiac catheterization was first put to practical use in 1941 by the French-American physiologist André Cournand, who won the Nobel Prize in 1956. Cardiac catheterization remains the basic technique of many invasive procedures for the diagnosis and treatment of heart disease.

The term "cardiac catheterization" in its early days was used to mean a specific, rather limited test consisting of the introduction of a catheter into the circulation, either through a vein into the right side of the heart and the pulmonary artery or through an artery into the aorta and the left side of the heart. The catheter permitted collecting blood samples from various parts of the circulation and measuring pressures in the heart and arteries. The earliest application of cardiac catheterization was in the diagnosis of some congenital heart diseases by showing abnormal communication between the two sides of the heart and abnormal pressures in the right side of the circulation. The original method involved making an incision in the skin and directly introducing the catheter into a vein under the skin. A simplified technique, called the percutaneous method, was first introduced in Sweden. It consists of puncturing a vein with a needle through the skin and introducing a wire through the needle. The needle is then withdrawn, and the catheter is slid into the vessel over the wire. This technique is particularly valuable in catheterizing an artery, a procedure that otherwise would require minor surgery (fig. 17). Percutaneous introduction of catheters into the blood vessels is now the basis for almost all invasive procedures, not only for diagnostic purposes but also for a variety of treatments of cardiovascular conditions. The most important application of this technique is in contrast cardiovascular radiology, particularly angiocardiography.

Cardiac catheterization as a general term now applies to a combined invasive diagnostic study involving several components. The goals of cardiac catheterization as an isolated procedure include

gathering basic hemodynamic data (cardiac output, intracardiac pressures) to evaluate the function of the two ventricles with the patient at rest and during mild exercise (pedaling a stationary bicycle during the procedure)

diagnosing pulmonary hypertension

determining pressure gradients between chambers (see chap. 7), which may indicate the severity of stenosis of cardiac valves

detecting abnormal communications between the two sides of the heart

Cardiac catheterization is almost always combined with angiocardiography, considered indispensable in reaching a diagnosis.

A special application of cardiac catheterization technique is hemodynamic monitoring of seriously ill patients in intensive-care or coronary-care units. This involves introducing into a vein a small catheter with an inflatable balloon near its tip. The balloon is then inflated, and the catheter is carried by the flow of venous blood into the right atrium, the right ventricle, and the pulmonary artery. This procedure does not require a cardiac laboratory or fluoroscopic facilities and can be performed in the intensive-care unit of a

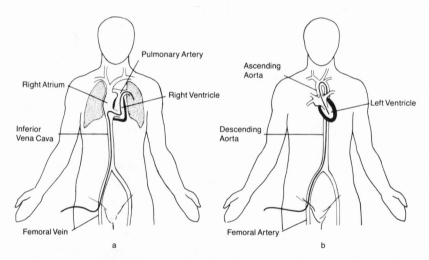

Figure 17. (a) The pathway of venous (right-sided) catheterization of the heart. The catheter enters the body via the femoral vein in the groin and is conducted through the inferior vena cava into the right side of the heart and hence into the pulmonary artery. (b) The pathway of arterial (retrograde) catheterization of the heart. The catheter is introduced into a femoral artery in the groin and is advanced (against the flow of blood) into the aorta and through the aortic valve into the left ventricle. The catheter can also be redirected, above the aortic valve, to enter the origin of each coronary artery in order to perform a coronary arteriogram.

hospital. The catheter can be left in place for several days, permitting continuous display of pressures inside the heart or pulmonary artery and intermittent determination of cardiac output.

Angiocardiography, or contrast radiography of the heart and blood vessels, is the most frequently performed study of the circulatory system and is used for examining other parts of the body as well (brain, kidney, lower extremities). It consists of introducing into the blood a liquid containing a radiopaque substance that shows up when photographed. Most tests require that the X-ray image be recorded on 35-mm film to appreciate the motion, although some tests require only still photographs. The contrast material used to be injected into the bloodstream through a vein, but it was found that the material became too dilute by the time it reached the parts of the circulation to be investigated. The standard technique now is to introduce the contrast material directly at the point of investigation by means of a catheter (*selective angiocardiography*).

Coronary arteriography is the most frequently performed invasive cardiac test. Special catheters are introduced into the large artery in the groin and guided into the aorta. The preformed catheter tips are conducted to the opening of each coronary artery as it leaves the aorta. A small amount of contrast material is injected directly into each, and the distribution of the opacified blood is recorded on 35-mm X-ray film. An alternate route for introducing the catheter into the arterial system is through the brachial artery (at the inside of the elbow).

Left ventriculography is the standard procedure for evaluating contractions of the left ventricle as well as calculating the ejection fraction (fig. 18) (see the discussion of nuclear ventriculography above, pp. 39–40). In patients undergoing coronary arteriography, a ventriculography is usually performed at the same time, since the data obtained by this method are more reliable than those obtained by the noninvasive technique.

Angiocardiography plays an important role in detecting congenital heart disease. In conjunction with cardiac catheterization, it allows the physician to diagnose some of the most complex lesions. It is also essential in evaluating disease of the cardiac valves by displaying valvular incompetence.

A refinement of angiographic technique is *digital subtraction angiography,* which enhances the faint image of opacified blood

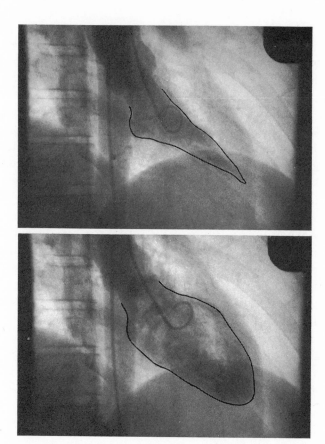

Figure 18. Two frames from a film showing the left
ventriculogram of a healthy person, performed by
injecting a contrast dye through a cardiac catheter into
the left ventricle. The upper frame (outline retouched)
shows the volume of the left ventricle at the end of
systole (lowest volume), the lower frame at the end of
diastole (highest volume). The difference between the two
volumes represents the amount of blood ejected into the
aorta by the recorded heartbeat. The volume of ejected
blood (stroke volume) divided by the highest volume in
diastole represents the percentage of blood pumped by a
heartbeat (the ejection fraction, in this example 84
percent), an important index of cardiac performance.

when the contrast substance is too dilute to be seen under ordinary radiography. This technique permits visualization of various parts of the vascular system after the contrast material is injected into a peripheral vein. This type of angiocardiography thus becomes a noninvasive procedure (intravenous injections are considered noninvasive). It provides clear pictures of the aorta and great vessels as well as somewhat limited images of the heart. Detailed viewing, however, still requires selective angiocardiography, particularly in visualizing the coronary arteries.

Another invasive diagnostic procedure indicated in special conditions is the *electrophysiological study.* Wires are introduced into various areas of the heart and record electrical potential directly from the inside of the heart. Such studies may also employ stimulation of the heart by an electronic pacemaker to observe responses of the heart and induce certain arrhythmias that reproduce those experienced previously by the patient.

Diagnosing Heart Disease

Present-day technology provides many sophisticated procedures for establishing a precise and correct diagnosis in a heart patient. The process of arriving at a diagnosis involves three steps: (1) history taking and physical examination, usually supplemented by electrocardiographic and radiographic examinations, (2) complex noninvasive tests, and (3) invasive tests. In a great many cases, step 1 may establish a reasonable diagnosis. Step 2 greatly increases the cost of the diagnosis; echocardiographic and nuclear studies range from five to ten times the cost of the electrocardiogram and chest X ray. Step 3 not only raises costs still further but also introduces an element of risk—the possibility of the test causing physical complications or even death. It should be noted that noninvasive tests are performed by technicians: the physician sees and interprets only the results of the test. Echocardiography and nuclear tests thus require a great deal of expertise from the technical staff before the physician reviews the findings. Invasive tests are in essence surgical procedures performed by cardiologists with special training supported by an expert team of nurses and technicians.

Interpreting test results presents two types of difficulties. First, tests aimed at establishing the presence of a certain abnormality do not always provide a definitive answer and may lead to a difference of opinion. Second, almost every test occasionally supplies incorrect information: certain changes expected to be present in a given disease may not be found (a false negative result), or the test may display changes suggesting a disease not present (a false positive result). In arriving at a diagnosis, the physician may encounter a maze of difficulties caused by uncertain, sometimes contradictory results of examinations and tests. Although establishing a correct diagnosis may represent a personal challenge to physicians, they should not lose sight of the goals of a detailed diagnosis: to determine the proper medical treatment for the patient and to evaluate the patient's prognosis. A diagnosis of heart disease can often involve much more testing than is necessary to fulfill these goals. Concerns about the cost of health care force us to consider the cost-benefit relationship that may lead to voluntary or imposed restrictions on performing tests, especially since cardiological procedures are among the most expensive in medicine.

Chapter Four

Treatment

Two kinds of treatment (therapy) of cardiac disease are generally recognized: (1) *preventive (prophylactic) therapy,* aimed at protecting a person from acquiring a disease or at halting the progress of existing disease, and (2) *remedial therapy,* aimed at abolishing or reducing symptoms or manifestations of a disease. Every intervention has to be considered from the standpoint of risk versus benefit to the patient. In this context risk is considered in a broad sense, including the possibility not only of death or worsening of health but also of unpleasant side effects or even undesirable changes in life-style.

The risk-benefit relationship applied to remedial therapy is clear-cut: every patient subjected to the risk of therapeutic intervention is expected to benefit from it; the implication is that if the goal of therapy is not attained, treatment is discontinued or changed. In preventive therapy the risk-benefit relationship is entirely different, because the benefit no longer can be gauged by the health of particular patients but rather is based on statistical probability. Many subjects are exposed to the risk—if there is any—but only a few are expected to benefit from the therapy. Consider these two examples. (1) If a certain population elects to modify its diet in the hope of reducing the probability of future heart attacks, the benefit cannot be measured; the risk, however, consists only of a voluntary change in life-style. (2) If anticoagulants are administered to patients who are known to be prone to form clots in the heart, in order to reduce the risk of a stroke, the drug introduces a different risk, though admittedly remote—that of a serious hemorrhage. Assume that for a certain group of cases the risk of stroke can be reduced by half—say, from one chance in 50 to one chance in 100. For each 100 patients, one will be spared the stroke—99 are subjected to risk of hemorrhage without expected benefit. Here a thoughtful consideration of the risk-benefit relationship is needed to decide in each case whether such treatment should be initiated.

Preventive cardiology is playing an increasingly important role in managing heart disease. Two types of prevention can be distinguished: (1) *primary prevention,* aimed at protecting a healthy person from developing a cardiac disease, and (2) *secondary prevention,* aimed at keeping disease already established in a patient from progressing or from leading to complications. The same type of intervention may be applied to primary and secondary prophylactic therapy. For example, institution of a low-fat, low-cholesterol diet is considered primary prevention, if applied to the general population, or secondary prevention, if applied to patients who have recovered from coronary heart attacks.

General Management of the Cardiac Patient

The majority of patients suffering from cardiac disease are afflicted by a chronic, often lifelong problem. Consequently, their medical management goes beyond conventional treatment and involves recommendations concerning life-style. Patients with milder varieties of heart disease are often permitted to lead a normal, totally unrestricted life, except for such minor interventions as administering an antibiotic drug before dental extractions as a precaution against infection. Children with heart disease may require specific instructions concerning physical education and recreational activities as well as vocational guidance. Patients whose disease have progressed to a point of some disability may need a detailed program regulating their activities and diet and may be counseled regarding some occupational and environmental factors.

The most detailed set of regulations applies to patients recovering from heart operations or from an acute myocardial infarction. Here a specially trained team may take charge of cardiac rehabilitation. The goal is to guide and facilitate the transition from acute hospital care to as normal a life as possible, while emphasizing secondary prevention of further heart damage. Cardiac rehabilitation is usually divided into three stages: stage 1 involves in-hospital treatment; stage 2, immediate convalescence; and stage 3, long-term support. During the first stage the patient is guided toward resuming activities at a gradual pace often by physical therapists and occupational therapists, in combination with psychological support. On leaving the hospital, the patient usually receives individual instruction regarding an exercise program, based on treadmill tests, as well as other advice regarding life-style. Exercise is often performed in organized rehabilitation units under medical supervision. The third stage is important for those patients who have some residual disability and may benefit from constant supervision.

Cardiac Drugs

Many drugs for the treatment of heart disease are now available, and the number is constantly increasing. Drugs are strictly regulated: new drugs can be placed on the market only after approval, following a series of tests, by the Food and Drug Administration. Three features of every drug are evaluated: (1) efficacy, (2) side effects, and (3) toxicity.

To demonstrate the effectiveness of a cardiac drug, controlled studies have to be performed. Typically its action is compared with that of a placebo, tablets similar in appearance to the drug but containing an inert substance, such as sugar. Inasmuch as responses to drugs vary from person to person, and some patients may even show improvement when taking the placebo (owing to psychological influences), large numbers of observations are often needed to demonstrate that a drug has the predicted effect on heart disease.

Side effects consist of undesirable consequences of taking a drug that may develop while the drug is administered in the recommended dose and exerting the desired effect on disease. Among common side effects of cardiac drugs are nausea, diarrhea, sleepiness, and reduced sexual drive.

Drug toxicity refers to serious, even fatal consequences of administering a drug. There are two mechanisms of drug toxicity: (1) toxic effect caused by a dosage that is too high for a given patient; and (2) toxic effect caused in certain patients who have or develop hypersensitivity to a certain drug even though it is being administered in the recommended dosage. Hypersensitivity to a drug often in-

volves allergic reactions that may become progressively more severe as treatment with the drug continues or when treatment is
repeated. Some of these reactions may be life-threatening.

Frequently treatment of a cardiac condition requires the administration of more than one drug. In that case it is necessary to take
into consideration the relationship of drugs to each other, or *drug
interaction*. In many instances two drugs have no such relationship:
each drug exerts its effect independently of the other. However,
drug interaction is common and may take place in a variety of ways:

Two drugs may facilitate each other's action, so that smaller doses of
each may attain the desired effect with better tolerance and
lower potential for toxicity (synergistic action).

Two drugs may reduce each other's potency, making higher doses
necessary to produce the desired effect (antagonistic action).

The addition of a second drug may alter the action of the first drug,
which may previously have been effective and well tolerated: the
new drug may make the first drug toxic in some instances or
simply ineffective in others.

Drug interactions are of considerable importance in patients requiring treatment by multiple drugs, and caution is required in select-
ing compatible drugs and regulating dosages.

Drugs are foreign substances the body tries to destroy or ex-
crete. Different drugs are handled in different ways: some are
eliminated with the urine or feces, some are destroyed by one of
the organs (usually the liver), and some are changed into inert
substances. The length of time it takes to eliminate an active drug
plays a role in the way the drug is administered. Most drugs are
absorbed from the gastrointestinal tract into the bloodstream,
where their level can be measured. Blood level of a drug decreases
at a fixed rate for each drug. The time required to halve drug
content in the blood from its initial level is called the half-life of a
drug, and it helps in determining how often a given drug has to be
taken by the patient. Most cardiac drugs have half-lives of a few
hours and hence must be administered at least three times a day.
Those with a long half-life need to be taken only once daily.

The standard method for administering cardiac drugs is in the
form of tablets or capsules. Liquid medicines are rarely used. How-

ever, for a variety of reasons drugs may have to enter the body by other than the oral route, or *parenterally.* Parenteral drug administration involves injecting the drug underneath the skin (subcutaneous), into a muscle (intramuscular), or into a vein (intravenous). A drug may be administered parenterally either because it acts faster thus administered than when given orally or because it would be destroyed by digestive juices.

In acutely ill patients parenteral administration of drugs is preferred. In such cases the most common means is continuous intravenous drip. The drug is dissolved in a solution of salt or glucose, and a measured amount enters the body, maintaining a steady level of the drug. By regulating the speed of the drip, the effect of the drug can be increased or decreased as the need arises. Other parenteral modes of administering drugs include *sublingual* (some drugs, such as nitroglycerin, take effect rapidly when dissolved under the tongue) and *transdermal* (some drugs can be absorbed through the intact skin as an ointment or on specially designed patches).

Drugs used specifically in the treatment of heart disease are categorized according to their pharmacological effects. Some drugs have multiple actions and are used for different purposes, such as for treatment of high blood pressure and of heart failure. In most categories there are several drugs with almost identical effects. Commonly used cardiac drugs can be grouped in two ways. The first is according to physiological action:

Drugs enhancing the force of cardiac contraction. The classic drug, digitalis, is derived from the foxglove plant and has been in continuous use for more than two hundred years. A few newer drugs are now available, predominantly for short-term treatment.

Diuretics. This widely administered group of drugs is used to counter fluid retention caused by heart failure and to treat hypertension.

Beta-adrenergic blocking agents. These drugs are capable of blocking one of the functions of the autonomic nervous system. The prototype of a drug in this category is propranolol, first developed in the 1960s. There are multiple uses of these drugs in heart disease—to reduce high blood pressure, to reduce or eliminate attacks of angina pectoris, to reduce or prevent certain arrhythmias, and to slow the heart rate.

Calcium channel blocking agents. These drugs relieve or prevent
spasm of blood vessels (particularly the coronary arteries), reducing high blood pressure, and reducing or eliminating attacks of
angina pectoris. In addition, several of these drugs have antiarrhythmic properties.

The second grouping is according to therapeutic effect:

Antiarrhythmic drugs. Drugs aimed at the prevention or elimination of arrhythmias include some drugs in the categories mentioned above. Quinidine and procainamide are the prototypes
and other powerful antiarrhythmic drugs have been introduced, some of them highly toxic but uniquely effective in life-
threatening arrhythmias.

Anti–heart failure drugs. Besides diuretics and drugs enhancing
the force of cardiac contraction, these include vasodilator drugs
that reduce the heart's workload and mitral regurgitation.

Antihypertensive drugs. Several categories of drugs have the property of reducing blood pressure, by various mechanisms. Treatment of hypertension thus often involves the use of more than
one drug, which together may act synergistically.

Antithrombotic drugs. The problem of clot formation within the
heart or the blood vessels is addressed by three types of drugs.
(1) Thrombolytic drugs, capable of dissolving existing clots. (2)
Drugs inhibiting aggregation of platelets in the blood, such as
aspirin, are used prophylactically. (3) Anticoagulant drugs are a
more effective means of clot prevention. However, they carry a
risk of bleeding and require periodic tests of their effectiveness.

Antianginal drugs. Nitrates (nitroglycerin and long-acting derivatives of it) dilate the coronary arteries. Other drugs include beta-
adrenergic and calcium channel blocking agents, both of which
act by reducing the requirements of the heart for oxygen.

Lipid-lowering drugs. These help reduce atherosclerosis by lowering the blood levels of cholesterol and triglyceride.

Drugs administered for remedial purposes need monitoring. In
some cases the effects are obvious to the physician or patient. For
instance, diuretics cause the patient to pass large quantities of

urine, and their effects can be measured by recording daily body weight. Antihypertensive drugs require frequent measurement of the blood pressure, which often can be done by the patient. The effectiveness of antianginal drugs is determined by the patient's observation regarding the number and severity of attacks of angina. In such cases the dosage of a drug and suitability of a particular therapy can be directly determined. Measurement of the blood content of some drugs may provide guidance in regulating dosages.

The effectiveness of drugs administered prophylactically cannot be evaluated directly. In some cases tests are available to help establish the dosage of a drug (for example, the prothrombin time test for anticoagulants) or to determine effectiveness (such as serum cholesterol level in the evaluation of cholesterol-reducing diets or drugs). If no tests are available to determine the safety of a prophylactic drug, a standard dosage is prescribed and maintained, provided no side effects develop.

Drug toxicity often presents serious problems. Immediate reactions in patients to a new drug can usually be controlled by reducing dosage or substituting a similarly acting drug. However, some cardiac drugs produce toxic reactions only after weeks or months of apparently successful treatment; furthermore, the toxic effect may not be apparent. Among such slowly appearing toxic effects are drug-induced reduction in white blood cells or platelets in the patient's blood, liver damage, development of cataracts, changes in personality, and depression. Some drugs have been suspected of being carcinogenic.

As stated, the potential toxicity of many cardiac drugs requires thoughtful consideration of the risks and benefits, especially in cases where a drug must be administered for long periods or permanently. Careful clinical observation and the performance of periodic blood and liver function tests may sometimes aid in detecting drug toxicity. Nevertheless, in certain life-threatening conditions, such as ventricular arrhythmias, the risk of serious toxic reaction is acceptable as a lesser evil.

Interventional Cardiac Therapy

Traditionally treatment of heart disease fit into two classes, medical and surgical. Now a third mode of treatment is available and widely used, intermediate between medical and surgical—*interventional therapy*, performed by specially trained cardiologists rather than cardiovascular surgeons. Some of these procedures represent alternatives to surgery; in selected cases they may be equally effective yet simpler and less expensive and require the patient to spend much less time in recovery. Others have specific uses and indications. Among such procedures are

balloon coronary angioplasty (percutaneous transluminal coronary angioplasty, or PTCA)

balloon valvuloplasty

temporary or permanent use of pacemakers

intraaortic balloon pump

interventional treatment of arrhythmias

Coronary angioplasty was developed in the late 1970s, and it has proven successful in relieving stenosis of the larger branches of the coronary arteries. Atherosclerosis of arteries produces plaques that reduce the amount of blood the artery is able to deliver to the affected organ. When such plaques significantly reduce the lumen of a coronary artery and are accessible, as demonstrated by coronary arteriography, angioplasty is performed by introducing a specially designed cardiac catheter into the arterial system. At one end of the catheter is a balloon, which when deflated fits snugly around the catheter; a separate channel connects it with the end of the catheter outside the body, through which it can be inflated. The inflated balloon has a long, cylindrical shape of fixed diameter, which can widen the tip of the catheter considerably, filling the inside of the artery. Under fluoroscopic examination the tip of the catheter is placed in the portion of the coronary artery narrowed by the plaque. The balloon is then inflated with a liquid at controlled and measurable pressure, compressing the plaque and thereby greatly reducing the stenosis (fig. 19). Cutting devices, lasers, and small framework-like devices called stents can be used in difficult cases.

The success of coronary angioplasty in improving blood supply to the heart by relieving obstruction in a coronary artery encouraged the development of a similar technique to relieve valvular narrowing. Balloon valvuloplasty works on the same principle as PTCA;

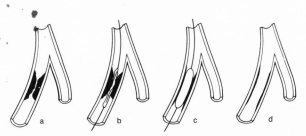

Figure 19. Coronary angioplasty. (a) Coronary branch showing severe stenosis. (b) Catheter placed in this branch with a deflated balloon at the level of the stenosis. (c) Inflated balloon compressing the stenosing plaques. (d) Minimal residual stenosis after the removal of the catheter.

the catheters and balloons are appropriately larger, and they differ in design. The catheter tip with deflated balloon is placed at the stenosed valve, which widens when the balloon is inflated.

Electronic pacemakers have been in use since the 1960s. They were introduced to provide protection from sudden death caused by failure of the natural pacemaker. The artificial pacemaker consists of a generator that rhythmically discharges electrical impulses. It is connected with an insulated wire inserted through the patient's venous system, so that its exposed tip is in contact with the muscle of the right ventricle or right atrium or both. The pacemaker has two functions: *pacing*, i.e. generating rhythmic electrical impulses, and *sensing*, i.e. detecting electrical impulses from the beating heart, which inhibit the artificial impulses from the generator. The sensing function permits the pacemaker to become active only when needed, assuming a standby function in patients who develop temporarily excessive slowing of the heart, or "pauses" (chap. 6). In patients with permanently slow heart rhythm the electronic pacemaker operates at all times. The point of stimulation of the heart is selected in accordance with the type of bradycardia (abnormally slow heartbeat): in diseases of the sinus node the atrium is stimulated; in complete heart block, the ventricle.

The pacemaker can be set up as a temporary measure, with the stimulating wire inside a cardiac chamber connected to a generator located outside the body. More often, however, pacing is permanent, in which case a miniaturized generator is placed under the skin in a small pocket made by surgical incision, usually underneath the collarbone. In permanent pacemakers the generator imbedded under the skin can be programmed from outside the body to adjust the heart rate.

Pacing has now become quite sophisticated. The most important development has been the *dual-chamber pacemaker.* Separate wires are introduced into the atrium and the ventricle. The generator can sense and initiate pacing of the atrium, if that chamber fails to receive the normal stimulus, or the ventricle, if the atrial impulse fails to reach the ventricle. Furthermore, if needed, both chambers can be sequentially paced, maintaining the natural interval between them.

Intraaortic balloon pumps act as boosters supporting the pumping action of a failing left ventricle. Inasmuch as such devices can safely be used for no more than a few days, this method of treatment is intended only to tide over a temporary malfunction of the left ventricle. A specially designed catheter is introduced into an artery in the groin and advanced into the descending aorta. The catheter is surrounded by an inflatable balloon along most of its length. The deflated balloon is connected to a pump (outside the body), which is synchronized with the heart action by means of signals coming from an electrocardiogram. During cardiac systole the balloon remains deflated; during diastole, when the aortic valves are closed, the pump inflates the balloon, which fills the inside of the aorta, thereby acting as a pump and displacing the blood (fig. 20). By this means the blood flow into the critical areas—the brain and the coronary circulation—receives an additional boost in diastole, supplementing the normal pumping action of the heart in systole; furthermore, this technique helps maintain blood pressure at an adequate level. The principal use of the intraaortic balloon pump is in the treatment of shock, particularly when it is caused by failure of a cardiac ventricle; it is also used in treating unstable angina pectoris (chap. 7) and in stabilizing some patients after open-heart surgery.

Interventional treatment of arrhythmias includes the following techniques:

external defibrillation of the heart in cardiac arrest

termination of tachycardias by electric shock (cardioversion) or by means of pacemakers deliberate induction of damage to the conducting system of the heart by means of special catheters to control certain life-threatening arrhythmias

Ventricular fibrillation, uncoordinated twitching of the heart muscle, is the commonest cause of cardiac arrest. The heart ceases to pump blood effectively, and the condition is fatal unless it can be reversed within four to five minutes. *External defibrillation*, application of electric current to the outside of the chest in the region of the heart by means of two conductive paddles, may restore normal heartbeat—the essential step in cardiac resuscitation.

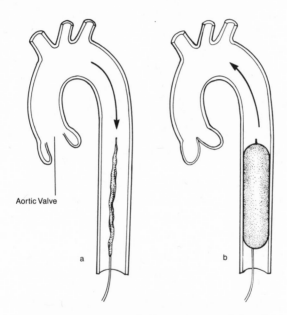

Aortic Valve

a   b

Figure 20. Intraaortic balloon pump. A deflated balloon is placed in the descending aorta and is connected with a pump, the action of which is synchronized with cardiac contraction and relaxation by means of an electrocardiographic signal. (a) During ventricular systole (open aortic valve) the balloon remains deflated and blood flow is normal. (b) During ventricular diastole (closed aortic valve) the balloon is inflated and displaces the blood in the descending aorta.

A related technique is used to restore a normal heart rhythm in certain arrhythmias involving *tachycardia,* abnormally rapid heart action. Here, however, the electric shock has to be delivered at a specific point in the cardiac cycle and must be synchronized by an electrocardiographic signal. This procedure, *cardioversion,* may be applied in emergencies for acute arrhythmias or electively for chronic arrhythmias. Whereas in cardiac arrest defibrillation is performed on unconscious patients, candidates for cardioversion, a very painful procedure, are conscious and hence have to be put under general anesthesia or heavy sedation.

A new application of the technique of treating arrhythmias electrically is the *implantable defibrillator and cardioverter,* which has been approved for limited use. At present this apparatus has to be inserted surgically, its wires sutured to the surface of the heart and its generator implanted under the skin. The objective of this method is to defibrillate automatically patients who develop ventricular fibrillation or to cardiovert ventricular tachycardia, thus preventing cardiac arrest. The generator is programmed to sense and diagnose ventricular fibrillation or ventricular tachycardia and to administer an appropriate electric shock to restore regular rhythm. The treatment is indicated only in patients with a clearly demonstrated high risk of fatal arrhythmia.

Certain tachycardias can be terminated by delivering rapid impulses by means of an electronic pacemaker placed temporarily with its tip in the right atrium. This method, *pacing overdrive,* is an alternative to cardioversion; it has the advantage of being painless, thus obviating the need for anesthesia.

A new method of treatment of certain serious arrhythmias originating in the atrium is now being developed and tested. Certain atrial arrhythmias occurring periodically may cause serious disability and be unresponsive to drug therapy. It is possible, by manipulating a specially designed catheter, to destroy the tract conducting impulses from the atria to the ventricles (the atrioventricular node or bundle of His), thereby shielding the ventricles from the rapid stimulation. Certain abnormal pathways can be destroyed while preserving the normal pathways. In some cases permanent pacemakers may be necessary after such an ablation procedure. Obviously, such a drastic step should be taken only if other means of controlling the heart fail.

Surgical Therapy

The development of heart surgery constitutes one of the most dramatic advances in the health field in this century. During most surgery on the heart today the pumping and oxygenating of the blood is done outside the body by a heart-lung machine. Few operations—resection of the pericardium, closed mitral valvotomy—can be performed on a beating heart with the blood circulating normally. Cardiopulmonary bypass is obligatory in open-heart surgery. There are four requirements for the performance of open-heart surgery: (1) the blood has to be pumped and oxygenated outside the body; (2) the heart cavities have to be empty; (3) the heart motion has to be stopped; (4) when the circulation and heart motion are restarted, the function of the ventricles has to be restored to its preoperative level.

When open-heart surgery was first developed in the 1950s, the task of fulfilling these requirements was indeed formidable. The pump-oxygenator was a highly complex apparatus; several units of blood were needed to start the procedure; and the rate of complications from the artificial perfusion alone was considerable. Since then technology has greatly simplified cardiopulmonary bypass. A simple pump-oxygenator services blood circulating outside the body in disposable tubes and containers (fig. 21). The heart is stopped by injecting into it a solution containing a combination of electrolytes (potassium is a major component). In addition, the heart is cooled so as to reduce its oxygen requirements (hypothermia). Present techniques attain almost perfect preservation of heart muscle function. Cardiopulmonary bypass surgery lasts from one to twelve hours, with some increase in risk in the longer operations. Although surgical results are usually related to the skill and experience of the cardiovascular surgeon, the overall success of the operation is greatly influenced by the contributions of the entire cardiac surgical team of physicians, nurses, and technicians, whose responsibility is to prepare the patient for surgery, administer general anesthesia, supervise the perfusion of blood during cardiopulmonary bypass, and attend to postoperative care.

The overall risk of heart operations varies widely. Several studies have shown that institutions performing a high number of operations are likely to have lower surgical mortality than other institutions.

Commonly performed heart operations include coronary bypass

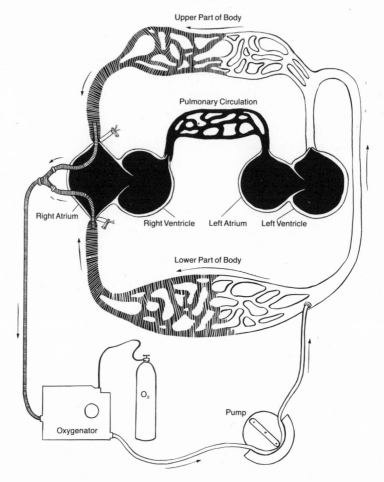

Upper Part of Body

Pulmonary Circulation

Right Atrium   Right Ventricle   Left Atrium   Left Ventricle

Lower Part of Body

O₂

Oxygenator

Pump

Figure 21. The artificial circulation used during open-heart surgery (cardiopulmonary bypass, using a heart-lung machine). Venous (deoxygenated) blood is
shown by shaded areas, oxygenated blood by white areas. Sections of the
circulation shown in black represent the areas bypassed by the artificial circuit
and void of blood, which can be opened for repair. All the blood returning
from the superior and inferior venae cavae is drained and channeled through
an oxygenator to be pumped into the arterial system. The blood is prevented
from reentering the heart by the closed aortic valve.

surgery, repair or replacement of heart valves, and correction of
congenital malformations of the heart. Coronary bypass is now the
most frequently performed major operation in the United States.
Even though it does not require opening the heart chambers, the
delicate suturing of the arteries has to be performed on a still heart.

Cardiac transplantation has now become a common operation. Its introduction in 1967 was followed by disillusionment because of the low survival rate. However, the development of effective drugs preventing rejection of the transplanted heart has successfully established this procedure, with the majority of patients surviving at least five years. The surgery itself is relatively simple, but the complexity of the overall subsequent care of transplant recipients limits its performance to a small number of institutions. Furthermore, the number of candidates for cardiac transplantation far exceeds the number of suitable donor hearts.

The *artificial heart* was widely publicized in the media in the mid-1980s when it was implanted into a few patients. Yet the dismal results and astronomical costs made it totally impractical. Some experts doubt whether it will ever become a viable form of treatment. However, a simple mechanical pump assuming the function of one or both ventricles has been used with some success as a temporary bridge when the heart fails totally, until a donor for cardiac transplantation becomes available.

Chapter Five

Performance of the Heart and Its Failure

The ultimate goal of the cardiac pump is to maintain sufficient circulation of blood to deliver oxygen to every cell of the body. The normal function of the heart requires a well-modulated contraction and relaxation of the cardiac muscle, at a rate between 50 and 80 beats a minute at rest, good coordination of the contractions of the atria and ventricles, and normal function of the four cardiac valves. Furthermore, the heart needs an adequate supply of fuel—oxygen—from the coronary circulation.

In addition to this central pump, the blood vessels and their content have an auxiliary role in maintaining blood pressure in the arterial system sufficient to supply blood to all organs. Furthermore, an adequate quantity of blood has to return to the heart via the venous system. The regulatory function of the blood vessels is acknowledged by the use of the term "peripheral pump" in referring to the contribution of blood vessels to cardiac performance.

These components of the circulation of blood are fine-tuned by a variety of reflexes and responses to signals arriving from the brain. Even change from rest to any type of activity requires major rearrangement of the circulation. The adjustment mechanisms operating in health are also responsible for adapting when some of the components malfunction.

The most important process of adaptation to abnormal conditions within the circulation is the response to increased workload. Normal cardiac reserve power can easily adjust to physical activity.

However, if the workload is unusually heavy, such as in professional athletes, the heart acquires additional strength by an increase in the size of its muscle fibers, a process called *hypertrophy* of the heart, analogous to the enlarging of the biceps in a weight lifter. The heart of an athlete usually weighs a little more than that of a sedentary person. However, this physiological hypertrophy has no known long-range deleterious effects on heart function.

In contrast to physiological hypertrophy of the heart, pathological hypertrophy can result from an involuntary increase in workload caused by significant abnormalities of the circulatory system. The difference between physiological and pathological hypertrophy lies in the amount of time the heart is exposed to the abnormal workload: an athlete spends only a small fraction of every 24 hours performing heavy work, whereas in pathological hypertrophy the overload is present continuously. Abnormal overload leads to more-pronounced hypertrophy of the heart, sometimes severe enough to double or even triple the weight of the heart. Pathological hypertrophy may bring about certain deficiencies in the delivery of oxygen to the heart muscle, which may eventually affect cardiac function and produce heart failure.

In accordance with the formula describing the work of the heart (a product of cardiac output and the pressure against which blood is ejected), increased workload may develop in one of two ways: (1) *pressure overload,* an increase in pressure within the arterial system (also referred to as systolic overload); or (2) *volume overload,* an increase in cardiac output (diastolic overload). Inasmuch as the left and right sides of the heart are pumps working independently (though synchronously), overload and the resulting hypertrophy can develop in either or both of the ventricles. Pressure overload of the left ventricle may be caused by severe hypertension (affecting the systemic circulation) or by narrowing of the outflow from the left ventricle (aortic stenosis). Pressure overload of the right ventricle can develop from increased pressure in the pulmonary circulation (pulmonary hypertension) or narrowing of the outflow from the right ventricle (pulmonary stenosis). Volume overload of the left ventricle may result from incompetence of left-sided cardiac valves (aortic regurgitation or mitral regurgitation); volume overload of the right ventricle occurs when certain congenital defects of the heart cause shunting of large amounts of blood from the left to the right side of the heart.

The development of compensatory hypertrophy of a cardiac ventricle is a slow and gradual process. It enables the patient to perform normally or near-normally and lead an active life, often unaware of the heart disease. The reduction of cardiac performance eventually producing heart failure occurs late, usually after many years of effective compensation.

Heart Failure

The term "heart failure" does not denote the fatal, terminal stage of heart disease but is customarily applied to any state in which the performance of the heart as a pump is significantly impaired. Heart failure means to the physician a set of symptoms and signs appearing in a patient whose heart is incapable of maintaining adequate circulatory function for supplying body tissues with oxygen under all circumstances. Such conditions may exist temporarily or permanently.

The left ventricle, which supports all tissues and organs with the exception of the lungs, is the principal area of the heart affected by cardiac disease. When functioning normally, it is capable of ejecting the needed amount of blood into the aorta with a normal filling pressure (less than 10 mm Hg). Impaired function of the left ventricle is present if the cardiac output (quantity of blood ejected) is less than normal or if higher diastolic filling pressure is required for ejecting blood. Since the left ventricular pressure is identical to the left atrial pressure during diastole, significant elevation of pressure in the left atrium and left ventricle during diastole acts as a dam, which has to be overcome by higher pressure in the veins, capillaries, and arteries of the lungs. Furthermore, the amount of blood in the lungs increases. This phenomenon is usually referred to as pulmonary congestion; the patient may sense stiffness in the lungs during respiration and experience shortness of breath (*dyspnea*). Rarely, if the malfunction of the contractile properties of the left ventricle develops abruptly, the capillaries of the lungs may permit an excess of fluid to enter the lungs, producing *pulmonary edema,* a life-threatening variety of dyspnea associated with coughing up frothy, bloody sputum.

The chain of events initiated by reduced performance of the left

ventricle begins during activities. A patient in the earliest stages of
heart failure is able to perform ordinary activities but becomes
short of breath during strenuous exercise he or she previously
tolerated. Further deterioration of ventricular function causes dyspnea in response to less-demanding activities. Eventually the tolerance of activities may become very limited, and dyspnea may appear without provocation, often at night.

The other effect of left ventricular malfunction, reduced cardiac
output, may be compensated for by tissues extracting more oxygen
from the blood, thus encroaching on the reserve. However, one
organ in the body is especially sensitive to a reduced blood
supply—the kidneys, the function of which includes regulating the
amount of salt and water in the body. They require a generous
blood supply; even a modest reduction of blood flow through the
kidneys may set in motion a mechanism involving certain hormones, which causes retention of salt and water.

In most cases of heart failure both increased filling pressure and
reduced cardiac output take place. High pressure accounts for most
of the symptoms, including dyspnea, and produces much of the
disability. Furthermore, high presssure in the pulmonary circulation may overload the right ventricle to a point where it begins to
malfunction. If this happens, high filling pressure in the right ventricle dams up the venous circulation returning the blood to the
heart from the tissues. This impairment in circulation may produce
enlargement of the liver and greatly increases the chance of fluid
retention, leading not only to more-pronounced swelling of the
lower extremities but also to accumulation of fluid in the chest
cavity (*pleural effusion*) and the abdominal cavity (*ascites*). The
lowered oxygen content of the blood in the tissues and the slowing
of the circulation may become visible through the vessels, giving
the skin or lips a bluish tint (*cyanosis*). Heart failure involving both
ventricles is referred to as congestive heart failure. When this is
present, the patient may experience severe weakness accompanying or replacing dyspnea. Sample pressure changes in heart failure
are shown in figure 22.

Patients' response to heart failure varies widely. The two principal consequences of it are dyspnea and fluid retention. Dyspnea
usually develops only in response to physical activity in the early
stages of heart failure. The discomfort related to shortness of breath

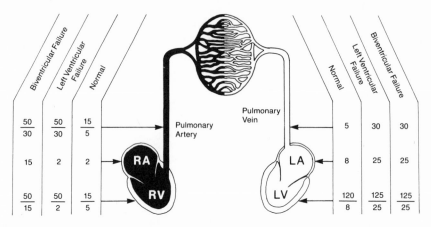

Figure 22. Examples of pressure changes in the heart and pulmonary circulation in left ventricular failure and in combined left and right ventricular failure.

during exercise can be avoided by reducing strenuous activity. Many patients do so intuitively and cease the activity before dyspnea appears; sometimes they are even unaware of their reduced tolerance for exercise, particularly if heart failure progresses very gradually. In most cases, however, patients become aware that activities hitherto easily performed can no longer be tolerated because of dyspnea, which leads them to seek medical care. In later stages dyspnea not only may appear without physical activity but also may be provoked by lying down, so that patients may have to sleep propped up in a half-sitting position (*orthopnea*) or may awaken at night from attacks of dyspnea or cough.

It should be emphasized that dyspnea is not specific to cardiac disease with heart failure but may also be produced by other conditions: a variety of diseases of the lungs, including pneumonia, emphysema, and tumors; spasm of the bronchi, such as occur during attacks of asthma; and accumulation of fluid in the pleural cavity. It may also develop in response to certain signals from the central nervous system, such as a reaction to anxiety.

Fluid retention manifests itself most frequently in swelling (*edema*) of the ankles, where fluid accumulates under the skin. More pronounced fluid retention shows up in the pleural and abdominal cavities and may cause considerable discomfort to the patient. However, heart failure is only one of several causes of edema.

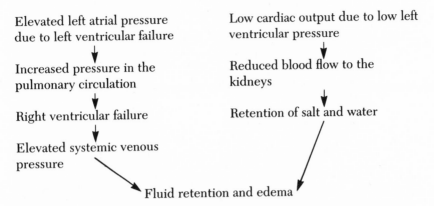

Figure 23. Two alternate mechanisms producing fluid retention and edema in heart failure.

There are three mechanisms involved in the accumulation of fluid (generally or locally): (1) *mechanical,* when pressure in the veins draining the legs or other areas is abnormally high; (2) *hormonal,* when the hormonal balance regulating salt and water is upset, such as occurs in reduced blood flow due to heart failure or in kidney disease; and (3) *osmotic,* when the protein content of the blood serum falls below a critical level, causing fluid to leave the capillary blood vessels. In heart failure, fluid retention in general and edema in particular are caused by mechanical and hormonal factors, as shown in figure 23. It should be noted, however, that abnormalities other than heart failure may also be responsible for edema: for example, edema of the lower extremities may result from an obstruction in the veins interfering with the return of blood from the legs.

Heart failure may develop abruptly (acute heart failure) or gradually, over a period of weeks, months, or years. The mechanisms of acute heart failure differ in patients with a previously healthy heart and circulation and those who already suffer from chronic heart disease. The former type involves a sudden severe injury, or insult, which cannot be compensated for by the cardiac reserve and its adaptive mechanism. It includes sudden overload of the heart or acute damage to the heart muscle. Left ventricular failure may develop after acute damage to one of the left cardiac valves (mitral or aortic regurgitation caused by an infection or trauma) or to the heart muscle (as in myocardial infarction). Right ventricular failure may result from increased pressure in the pulmonary artery caused by a large *thrombus* (clot) traveling to the lung and obstructing the flow of blood. Acute heart failure in patients who suffer from a chronic cardiac illness but are able to lead a normal or near-normal life is almost always preceded by some event affecting the heart or circulation: cardiac arrhythmia, as the onset of atrial fibrillation; new damage to the heart muscle, such as an acute coronary episode; or problems affecting the patient as a whole, such as infection, trauma, surgery, and failure of a major organ (kidney, liver, etc.).

Chronic cardiac failure is usually the end result of prolonged heart disease producing either persistent cardiac overload or damage to the heart muscle. Common causes of chronic overload include severe hypertension, valvular heart disease, and congenital cardiac malformations. Causes of myocardial disease include coronary-artery disease and cardiomyopathy.

As a rule, gradual development of heart disease is characterized by long periods during which the patient may lead a normal, unrestricted life. Deteriorating function of the heart may only be detectable by special tests, such as echocardiography or radionuclide studies. Disabling symptoms, particularly dyspnea, may progress very slowly: it is often difficult to pinpoint the onset of heart failure. The great majority of patients with heart failure—in both its acute and chronic varieties—responds to treatment, which can reduce or even totally eliminate disability. Depending on the nature and severity of cardiac disease, successful medical or surgical therapy of heart failure can prolong life or at least make life more tolerable.

Treatment of Heart Failure

The approach to treatment of heart failure involves applying several principles, depending on its cause and severity:

elimination of the overload primarily responsible for heart failure

improvement of the contractility of the heart muscle

elimination of excess fluid

reduction of cardiac workload by lowering arterial pressure or decreasing the volume of blood returning to the heart

Eliminating or ameliorating the disease that overloaded the heart and eventually led to its failure is the most effective treatment, though only a small number of cases is suitable for this approach. Successful medical or surgical treatment not only can improve the patient's condition but can even cause a gradual regression of cardiac hypertrophy, as shown by appropriate changes in the electrocardiogram and echocardiogram.

To increase the strength of contraction of the failing heart, digitalis and its derivatives are the traditional drug of choice. They can be administered intravenously for acute heart failure and orally over long periods. Several new drugs, administered by injection, have now been introduced; they can produce effective short-term improvement in cases of acute heart failure. At the present time several drugs capable of stimulating cardiac performance when taken orally are being tested. Their long-term safety and effectiveness are as yet uncertain.

Treatment aimed at controlling fluid retention involves two steps. In milder cases restriction of salt intake in the diet may effectively prevent fluid retention and restore prefailure cardiac function. In the majority of cases, however, diuretic drugs provide the most effective treatment for heart failure. Administration of diuretics has an immediate effect and often leads to a dramatic improvement of a patient's condition by controlling dyspnea and eliminating the consequences of fluid retention. It should be noted that fluid retention not only causes symptoms that produce discomfort but also affects unfavorably the function of the heart by inducing some overload, which can be eliminated by diuretic therapy. Such treatment often permits the patient to lead an active life even though the function of the cardiac pump may be permanently impaired.

In the 1970s an extremely effective group of drugs capable of reducing the workload of the heart was introduced. These drugs are known as vasodilators, or afterload reducers. This treatment works either by lowering the blood pressure or by reducing the resistance that the heart pumps against. It differs from the elimination of overload in that the latter treatment is capable of restoring normal function, whereas the former merely lowers the normal workload. When cardiac workload is reduced, regardless of the cause of heart failure, symptoms may be successfully controlled. This treatment is now widely used in patients with congestive heart failure.

The principal goal of treatment of heart failure is to alleviate symptoms and improve the life-style of patients suffering from serious heart disease. Only treatments successfully correcting the cause of failure, such as surgical correction of valve diseases or management of hypertension, can be considered to cure congestive heart failure. Vasodilator drugs, however, do reduce the annual mortality rate in chronic heart failure. It has not been definitively established whether medical therapy in chronic heart failure not amenable to direct intervention prolongs life.

The need for medical therapy varies widely. In many patients, particularly those with acute heart failure, treatment may be discontinued as the patient recovers from an episode of cardiac failure. In milder cases of chronic heart failure dietary restriction or occasional use of diuretics may be the only treatment needed. In some cases continuous therapy using one or more drug is essential if the patient is to obtain the full benefit of the therapy. There remain patients who are severely disabled despite the best available treatment. These patients have what physicians term end-stage heart failure and are potential candidates for the treatment of last resort, namely, cardiac transplantation.

Chapter Six

Arrhythmias

The healthy heart has a regular sequence of action. The process of impulse formation and its conduction from the pacemaker to the ventricles has been described in chapter 2. The regularity of the heartbeat, its rate, and the origin and spread of impulses all can deviate from the norm. The general term covering these abnormalities, regardless of their origin or significance, is *arrhythmia,* or disturbance of heart rhythm. The term is used even if the rhythm, or regular sequence of beats, is undisturbed but the rate is too slow or too fast.

The normal heartbeat is carefully regulated. At rest the rate is kept within relatively narrow limits, between 50 and 80 beats a minute in adults. During excitement and exercise the heart rate rises. The highest rate attained during strenuous exercise is between 160 and 200 beats a minute. The rhythm, under normal circumstances, is called *sinoatrial rhythm* (since it originates at the sinoatrial node) or *sinus rhythm.* It is customary to limit applying this term to moderate rates in the range of 50 to 100 beats a minute. When the heart rate exceeds 100 beats a minute, it is referred to as rapid rate, or *tachycardia,* regardless of whether it represents a normal phenomenon (such as during exercise) or an abnormal one. Conversely, a rate below 50 beats a minute is called slow rate, or *bradycardia.* Slow or rapid rate may originate in the normal pacemaker (sinus bradycardia and sinus tachycardia) or may be a manifestation of an abnormal rhythm. Abnormal ranges of impulse formation in the S-A node, when not caused by such factors as exercise, are usually related to signals from the autonomic nervous system and are more often manifestations of disturbances outside the heart than of heart disease. For example, tachycardia can accompany fever or shock; bradycardia may be associated with fainting or nausea.

The normal rhythm of the heartbeat is almost perfectly regular. There are times, however, when an irregularity of the rhythm is entirely due to a normal variation of the firing sequence in the S-A node. Such irregularities are called *sinus arrhythmias* and are usually related to the breathing, such as slight slowing of the rate during inspiration of air and slight speeding during expiration. It is especially common in children.

It is important to recognize that these normal variants—sinus bradycardia, sinus tachycardia, and sinus arrhythmia—do not represent real disturbances of the heartbeat. Identification of their normal mechanism can be made with the aid of the electrocardiogram. They should not be confused with real disturbances of cardiac rhythm, which are customarily divided into abnormalities of impulse formation and abnormalities of impulse conduction.

The Mechanism of Arrhythmias

The heart contains other pacemakers than the S-A node, and they serve as emergency backup. These are the secondary pacemaker located in the A-V node and the tertiary pacemaker located in the cells of the Purkinje system (see chap. 2). Under certain conditions cells of other parts of the conducting system connecting the A-V node with both ventricles are able to initiate electrical stimulation of the heart; furthermore, most ordinary muscle cells, the role of which is contraction and relaxation, may under abnormal conditions take on the role of pacemaker. Ordinarily the secondary and tertiary pacemakers kick in only if an impulse from above fails to arrive; such single heartbeats or series of beats are said to be activated by default; they are referred to as *escape beats*, and a series of them represent an *escape rhythm*. However, these reserve pacemakers may assume an active role and discharge an electrical impulse out of turn, before the expected stimulation from above arrives. Such premature single impulses are called *ectopic beats*, and groups of them are called *ectopic rhythms;* they represent abnormal stimulation of the heart by usurpation (figs. 24–25).

Ectopic beats or rhythms may originate at any point of the con-

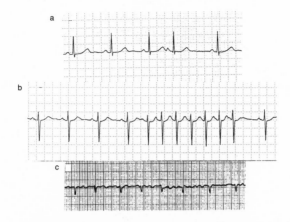

Figure 24. Atrial arrhythmias exemplified by strips of single electrocardiographic leads. (a) Premature (ectopic) atrial beat (no. 4). (b) A short run (paroxysm) of atrial tachycardia (seven beats). (c) Atrial fibrillation: there are no P waves, only rapid and irregular atrial deflections; the response of the ventricular complexes is totally irregular.

ducting system or even in abnormally stimulated heart muscle cells. Impulses originating in the upper part of the conducting system, including the A-V node, are termed *supraventricular;* their appearance in the electrocardiogram is identical with that of normal beats, as their impulses are transmitted along normal pathways to the ventricle, causing its depolarization and initiating its contraction. Ectopic impulses originating in the lower portion of the conducting system are called *ventricular* beats or rhythms. These impulses stimulate the ventricle in an abnormal sequence, which expresses itself in the electrocardiogram by wider, abnormal QRS complexes and T waves (fig. 25a).

Sequential ectopic beats are almost always at a faster than normal rate, that is, are ectopic tachycardias (supraventricular or ventricular). Supraventricular tachycardia can usually, though not always, be identified by electrocardiography as either atrial or junctional (A-V nodal) in origin. Occasionally it is associated with impulses traveling to the ventricle along abnormal pathways, shown in the electrocardiogram as wide complexes similar to those present in ventricular tachycardia.

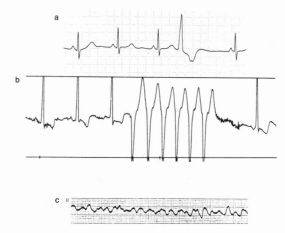

Figure 25. Ventricular arrhythmias exemplified
by strips of single electrocardiographic leads. (a)
Premature ventricular beat. (b) A short run
(paroxysm) of ventricular tachycardia (seven
beats). (c) Ventricular fibrillation: chaotic, small,
rapid complexes incapable of maintaining
coordinated heartbeat produce cardiac arrest.
Note that ventricular complexes in a and b are
broader than, and differ in shape from, normal
complexes.

　　　Abnormal activity of designated pacemaker cells or stimulated
myocardial fibers is not the only mechanism for the origin of
ectopic beats or ectopic rhythms. The alternative mode of production of arrhythmias is *reentry*, a phenomenon to which an important arrhythmogenic role has been attributed. To explain the concept of reentry, it is necessary to recapitulate some facts of normal
electrophysiology. The cardiac conducting system transmits electrical impulses sequentially from the S-A node through the atrium to
the A-V node, then along the bundle of His and its branches to the
ventricles. This basically unidirectional conducting system is capable of conducting impulses in the reverse direction as well, though
this does not take place under normal conditions. However, in the
presence of arrhythmias impulses activating the ventricles may first
send signals back to the atria, so that atrial contraction follows
ventricular contraction. All cardiac cells (contractile myocardial
cells as well as conducting fibers) have a *refractory period:* immedi-

ately after a cell's designated function (contraction or conduction) is completed, there is a short time in which they do not respond to stimulation. The refractory period accounts for the fact that once the impulse reaches its final destination, it cannot travel backward. However, if there is an abnormal slowing within any portion of the conducting system (including its final pathway inside the ventricular muscle), the impulse may be reactivated when conduction is already responsive after the refractory period is over. The reactivated impulse may stimulate the ventricle into an additional (premature) contraction, an *echo beat,* and may travel forward or backward to any part of the heart, producing various arrhythmias.

An echo beat represents the simplest kind of reentry. More complex situations arise when the relationship between velocity of conduction forward and backward permits impulses to travel back and forth at regular, rapid rates (most frequently between 180 and 250 beats a minute), producing reentry tachycardia. Both supraventricular tachycardia (featuring narrow QRS complexes in the electrocardiogram) and ventricular tachycardia (featuring broad complexes) can be caused by reentry.

The electrocardiographic appearance of arrhythmias produced by abnormal impulse formation and that caused by reentry are almost identical and cannot always be differentiated. Yet such a differentiation can be of some practical importance because certain drugs may control one mechanism but not the other. Furthermore, certain varieties of reentry arrhythmias have been successfully treated by surgery.

More-advanced disturbances of the cardiac rhythm are *flutter* and *fibrillation* of the atria or the ventricles. The mechanism of these arrhythmias is somewhat similar to reentry: the electrical impulse is never extinguished but travels continuously through the affected portion of the heart. *Atrial flutter* produces a rapid, regular response, usually at a rate of 300 beats a minute, initiating a weak contraction of the atrial muscle. Because of their refractory period the ventricles are unable to respond to each atrial contraction, only to every other impulse (hence the ventricular rate is usually about 150 beats a minute, and the rhythm is regular). *Atrial fibrillation* occurs when the impulse travels through the atria at still-faster rates, leading to a chaotic twitching of the atrial muscle, which no longer can contract. The ventricles respond only to some of the more powerful impulses and in an irregular fashion. The ventricular rate in atrial fibrillation (not influenced by drugs) is usually between 150 and 180 beats a minute, and its rhythm is totally irregular (fig. 24c). Flutter and fibrillation also affect the ventricles. But whereas the cardiac function can be maintained despite a weak or absent atrial contraction, ventricular fibrillation or flutter is tantamount to cessation of the circulatory function of the heart—cardiac arrest.

Disorders of Cardiac Conduction

The process of conducting impulses through the heart can be disturbed in three ways: (1) by a delay at a given point, (2) by its total interruption somewhere along the pathway, and (3) by nonresponsiveness of some part of the pathway.

Abnormal delay in conduction usually occurs between the atria and the ventricles, presumably because something slows the transit of the impulses through the A-V node. Such a delay is shown in the electrocardiogram by the fact that the interval between the P wave and the QRS complex is prolonged beyond the normal 0.2 seconds. This phenomenon is called *first-degree heart block* or *first-degree A-V block* (fig. 26b). First-degree heart block does not disturb the rhythm or the rate of the heart. It is primarily detected by the electrocardiograph. Its importance lies in demonstrating that the patient's conducting system is imperfect, and it may precede more serious forms of conduction disturbances.

A higher degree of impairment of conduction between the atria and the ventricles is a *second-degree heart (A-V) block,* a condition in which a certain number of impulses from the atria never reach the ventricle (figure 26c). Thus, one out of every two or more impulses from the atria is lost, producing dropped beats. The result may be an irregular heart action (if dropped beats occur every third beat or more) or a regular rhythm (if every other beat is dropped, *two-to-one heart block*).

The next level of disturbance of atrioventricular conduction is its total interruption, *third-degree heart (A-V) block,* also called *complete heart (A-V) block.* Here the atria and the ventricles act entirely independently of each other: the atria contract as a result of the normal S-A mechanism; the ventricles contract as a result of a

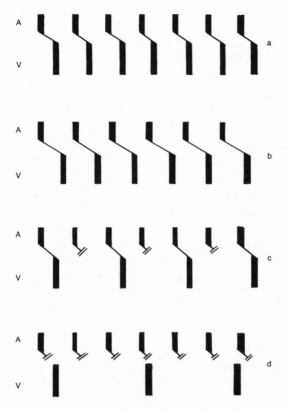

Figure 26. Diagram showing the sequence of
beats under normal conditions and in various
forms of heart block. The upper bar (A)
represents atrial depolarization, the lower bar
(V) ventricular depolarization. The oblique line
joining the 2 bars is the atrioventricular
conduction.

a. Normal conduction.

b. First-degree heart block showing a delayed
atrioventricular conduction, hence a longer
interval between the contraction of the atria and
the ventricles.

c. Second-degree heart block, showing every
other beat blocked and prevented from reaching
the ventricle. The ventricular rate is one-half
that of the atria.

d. Complete heart (A-V) block. All
communication between the atria and the
ventricles is interrupted. Consequently, the atria
and the ventricles beat independently of each
other, the ventricular rate usually much slower
than the atrial rate.

ventricular pacemaker with a slow rhythm unrelated to the atrial activity (fig. 26d). In complete heart block the atria usually maintain the normal heart rate of 70 beats a minute; the ventricles beat only 30 to 40 times a minute. This unusually slow ventricular rate imposes obvious problems on the maintenance of the circulation. In an otherwise sound heart the circulation can be maintained reasonably well, especially if the patient's activities are restricted; in the presence of serious heart disease such a low rate may precipitate heart failure. However, the principal danger of complete heart block lies in the fact that the ventricular pacemaker constitutes the last line of defense: its failure leaves the heart without any impulses, hence without contraction. Such failure of the ventricular pacemaker occasionally occurs in complete heart block for short periods (less than two minutes), causing loss of consciousness, and is known as *cardiac syncope* or *Stokes-Adams attack*. The danger of such an attack is self-evident: if it lasts more than four minutes, the patient will die.

The three degrees of heart block may be temporary or permanent. Temporary heart block may be due to acute, reversible illness, to the action of drugs, or to nervous influences; permanence implies complete, organic destruction of a given part of the conduction pathway.

If the interruption of conduction pathways occurs in the section below where the bundle of His divides into two branches, the impulse reaches the ventricle through the healthy bundle, so that the rhythm of the heart is not disturbed. However, if one of the ventricles fails to receive the impulses directly from the conduction pathways and the other ventricle is activated via a detour, the second ventricle contracts with a slight delay. This delay does not necessarily affect the function of the heart, but it causes gross distortion of the electrocardiogram. This type of conduction defect is called *bundle-branch block* (right or left, depending on which bundle is damaged). Bundle-branch block is a common disorder in some forms of heart disease, particularly in diseases of the coronary arteries.

Disturbances of the conduction system due to nonresponsiveness of the conducting tissues has already been touched on in connection with atrial flutter and fibrillation, in which not all rapid impulses can reach the ventricles. Other conditions in this category include *atrioventricular dissociation,* a disorder in which the A-V node fires at an abnormally high speed, faster than the S-A node, and therefore takes priority in activating the ventricles. Nonresponsiveness of conducting pathways may separate these impulses from the atria, which obey the normal S-A node stimulation. This situation resembles complete heart block in that the atria and the ventricles beat independently of each other, although here, by contrast, the atrial rate is usually slower than the ventricular rate. Such conditions are almost always temporary, usually do not last long, and often reflect the influence of factors outside the heart (drugs or a disturbance of salt and water metabolism).

Significance and Consequences of Arrhythmias

The function and efficiency of the cardiac pump under ordinary circumstances is not affected if the rhythm becomes irregular: the heart can adapt to an irregularity, even to the absence of effective atrial contraction. Arrhythmias frequently affect normal hearts in healthy individuals: monitor studies have shown that single ectopic beats can be found in almost one-half of the general population. Occasionally, healthy subjects display groups of ectopic beats (short runs of tachycardia), and even more complex arrhythmias sometimes appear. However, arrhythmias are more frequent in patients with heart disease and may produce serious consequences. The importance of arrhythmias in general is in its effect on cardiac function, its relationship to the underlying disease, and its role as a harbinger of life-threatening arrhythmias.

The function of the heart may be compromised if the heart rate is very fast or very slow. Tolerance of rapid tachycardia or slow bradycardia varies from person to person: in healthy populations only extremes in heart rate are likely to affect cardiac function; patients with cardiac disease, however, may be sensitive even to a moderate increase or decrease in heart rate, which may have serious consequences. The more common instances of arrhythmias in patients with organic heart disease, as already mentioned, may be an unimportant by-product of the underlying disease. But in some cases arrhythmias may accentuate the symptoms of the disease and affect cardiac function; in still others they may produce cardiac emergencies.

Perception of arrhythmias as palpitations is one of the symptoms that lead patients to seek medical care. As such, they may be a clue to the discovery of previously unknown, significant cardiac disease. Both healthy individuals having arrhythmias and patients with cardiac disease may be aware of the irregularity of their heartbeat. Even simple premature ectopic beats are often perceptible: ectopic ventricular beats usually cancel the next normal beat, producing a longer than usual pause that the affected person can feel as a skipping of heartbeats. Tachycardias often are perceived as palpitations or pounding of the heart. Yet some people, with or without heart disease, may be totally unaware of even the most complex arrhythmias.

Ventricular arrhythmias are potentially more serious than atrial arrhythmias, even though they are common in healthy persons. Since the most severe variety of ventricular arrhythmia is fibrillation—that is, cardiac arrest—some such arrhythmias need to be carefully studied to determine whether the patient is at a high risk of developing a fatal arrhythmia and thus requires aggressive treatment.

Common Arrhythmias

Paroxysmal atrial (supraventricular) tachycardia is characterized by sudden onset (perceived almost always as a pounding of the heart) and abrupt, spontaneous termination. It can last from minutes to several days. It often affects young, healthy persons: in some, attacks may recur only at long intervals; other may remain susceptible to frequent attacks, which can produce periodic disability. Many tachycardias respond to various maneuvers applied by a physician or even by patients themselves. These include applying pressure to the carotid artery in the neck, holding one's breath, or straining to force respiration, any of which may terminate an attack. Intravenous administration of certain drugs is more reliable in restoring normal heart rhythm. In rare instances, particularly when the rapid rate is poorly tolerated by the patient and unresponsive to drug therapy, it may be necessary to administer direct-current electric shock (cardioversion). As a general rule, no treatment of paroxysmal atrial tachycardia is needed between attacks; but if attacks recur frequently, preventive drugs can be prescribed.

Atrial flutter and atrial fibrillation are the most serious disruptions of atrial rhythm. These two arrhythmias are related and may occur in the same patient. Both may develop in healthy persons but are more frequent in patients with various cardiac disorders. Atrial flutter and atrial fibrillation can be paroxysmal, that is, terminate within hours or days, or permanent, in which case normal rhythm usually should be restored by various interventions.

As mentioned, in atrial flutter the rhythm is regular and the heart rate (rate of ventricular contractions) is about 150 beats a minute since the ventricles respond to alternate atrial impulses. Drugs can partially block the pathways to every third impulse, reducing the rate to 100 beats a minute, or to every fourth impulse, lowering the rate to 75 beats a minute, thereby abolishing the tachycardia. Atrial flutter can in most cases be terminated by one of three methods: drugs, electric shock, or pacemaker stimulation of the right atrium (see chap. 4).

Atrial fibrillation is a much more common arrhythmia than atrial flutter; in fact, it is one of the most frequently encountered arrhythmias, particularly in patients over 60 years of age. Before the start of treatment the ventricular rate is usually within the range of 150 to 180 beats a minute, and the rhythm is irregular. Atrial fibrillation may develop as a complication of many cardiac disorders but most often results from mitral stenosis. The rapid rate of untreated atrial fibrillation, its major deleterious effect, is often poorly tolerated and may induce heart failure. Even in otherwise healthy persons atrial fibrillation may produce considerable discomfort, although it is unlikely to affect cardiac function. The rapid heart rate can be promptly and predictably reduced by drugs to a rate comparable to that of a normal, though irregular, rhythm, thereby alleviating the discomfort and other consequences. With a heart rate adequately controlled by a program of drug therapy, a patient may remain in atrial fibrillation for years and lead an active life. Thus atrial fibrillation is not a life-threatening arrhythmia. However, it does introduce a serious risk: the noncontracting atria can facilitate the development of blood clots attached to their walls, which can break loose and travel within the arterial system, producing emboli (clots occluding important vessels) and leading in some cases to stroke.

The approach to the treatment of atrial fibrillation involves two options: restoring normal rhythm or slowing the heart rate in patients remaining in atrial fibrillation. Normal rhythm can almost always be restored either by drugs or by cardioversion. Restoration of normal rhythm is obviously the more advantageous option. But in patients prone to atrial fibrillation the arrhythmia may recur despite a course of preventive drugs. Patients who remain in atrial fibrillation are often given anticoagulants, drugs that inhibit clot formation, as protection against stroke. The choice of restoration of normal rhythm or control of the ventricular rate is usually made after estimating the probability of the arrhythmia recurring, which in turn may depend on the underlying cardiac disease.

Ventricular arrhythmias present one of the most difficult problems in cardiology. On the one hand, ventricular arrhythmias are ubiquitous in healthy adults; on the other hand, they can eventually result in fatal ventricular fibrillation. Consequently, a great deal of attention is given to recognizing and classifying them. Furthermore, ventricular arrhythmias are often closely linked to serious diseases of the myocardium, as evidence of electrical instability (the tendency to develop serious arrhythmias), and then require aggressive intervention.

Whereas the clinical importance of ventricular arrhythmias primarily depends on the underlying condition of the heart muscle, their appearance in the electrocardiogram often provides clues as to their prognostic significance. The simplest ventricular arrhythmia is the ventricular premature (ectopic) beat. However, its shape and timing in relation to the preceding normal beat may be telling. Ventricular ectopic beats that are alike and fixed in their timing are the least significant, except when they occur before the T wave of the preceding beat is completed. Ectopic beats varying in shape and timing may be evidence of electrical instability. Ectopic beats appearing in pairs or in groups of three are also considered potentially more serious. Ventricular ectopic beats appearing in runs of more than three beats are called ventricular tachycardia. All varieties of ventricular arrhythmia, including short runs of ventricular tachycardia, may be present in healthy persons; however, the more precarious the type of arrhythmia, the higher the probability of an underlying heart problem. Simpler ventricular arrhythmias do not affect heart function or cause discomfort.

Ventricular tachycardia plays a pivotal role in the evaluation of arrhythmias and in decisions regarding management, for under certain circumstances it can degenerate into fatal ventricular fibrillation. Ventricular tachycardia is usually similar to supraventricular tachycardia in its effect on the circulation and in discomfort to the patient, but its prognostic implications are different. It is customary to classify ventricular tachycardia into two types, *nonsustained* and *sustained*. The former is characterized by spontaneous resumption of normal rhythm; the latter persists until terminated by intervention. Nonsustained tachycardia may not compromise health; sustained tachycardia is always considered serious. Ventricular flutter and ventricular fibrillation are the commonest causes of cardiac arrest. As a rule, ventricular fibrillation is fatal unless treated immediately. Occasionally, however, ventricular flutter and fibrillation appear in nonsustained form, and normal rhythm spontaneously resumes in less than four minutes, in which case they result in cardiac syncope (see chap. 7).

Evaluation of ventricular arrhythmias requires two steps: recognition of the type and frequency of arrhythmia and diagnosis of its cause, including any underlying heart disease. An ordinary electrocardiogram is inadequate for diagnosing the extent of the arrhythmia. For that purpose it is necessary to record a continuous electrocardiographic tracing by means of a Holter monitor, which can display every heartbeat over a 24-hour period. An alternate method is continuous electrocardiographic monitoring of patients in an appropriate unit in a hospital; important arrhythmias observed on the video display are then printed out for further examination.

In evaluating the background of the arrhythmia, the physician considers the state of the heart, especially the presence of heart disease, and the possible specific causes of arrhythmias, such as acute myocardial infarction, myocardial ischemia, the toxic effect of a drug, abnormalities of electrolytes or acid-base balance, and certain abnormalities of renal or hepatic function. If the ventricular arrhythmia is of a serious variety and none of the reversible causes can be identified, except for the presence of myocardial disease, further tests may be indicated, including an electrophysiological study. Here the patient is taken into a cardiac catheterization laboratory, where a pacing wire is introduced into a cardiac ventricle. The heart can then be stimulated through the wire by an electronic pacemaker outside the body to determine whether an appropriate stimulus can initiate a nonsustained or sustained ventricular tachycardia. Such pacing studies can also be used for testing responses to antiarrhythmic drugs. In patients in whom the pacing stimulus induces a ventricular tachycardia, stimulation is repeated after a drug is administered: if tachycardia can no longer be induced, the drug may be considered efficacious in preventing naturally occurring attacks. However, there is still some controversy as to whether suppression of artificially induced tachycardia translates into reliable prevention of future attacks.

Treatment of ventricular arrhythmias includes both prophylactic and remedial therapy. The latter is rather limited, involving emergency treatment of ventricular tachycardia and ventricular fibrillation, termination of tachycardias, and the elimination of frequent premature beats that may produce discomfort or disability. Prophylactic therapy is the principal goal of antiarrhythmic treatment and includes a wide range of approaches. The most important caution in initiating prophylactic therapy of ventricular arrhythmia is that antiarrhythmic drugs carry a definite risk to the patient. Some have undesirable side effects that may unfavorably affect quality of life; furthermore, drugs may compromise the function of vital organs such as the blood, liver, and kidneys. And in about 10 percent of patients arrhythmias could be made worse by such drugs, owing to a paradoxical action. Thus the physician has to balance the risk of antiarrhythmic therapy against the risk of serious arrhythmias developing in the future. Short-range antiarrhythmic therapy, such as may be indicated in acute myocardial infarction, presents no problem; but the persistence of ominous arrhythmias may require lifelong antiarrhythmic therapy, which—particularly in patients who have no symptoms—poses a serious dilemma as to whether and when treatment is indicated. In the minority of cases successful treatment may be accomplished if a clear cause of ventricular arrhythmias can be identified and eliminated.

In general, certain priorities are assigned in initiating antiarrhythmic therapy. The first priority is given to patients who have been resuscitated from cardiac arrest. Second, aggressive therapy is usually needed for patients with recurrent sustained ventricular tachycardia. Last, patients with less-serious ventricular arrhythmias are often grouped according to the precariousness of the observed arrhythmias and the severity of underlying heart disease. Those with no evidence of organic heart disease usually require no treatment; those with myocardial disease are treated aggressively, particularly if myocardial function is seriously impaired. During the 1980s a large number of new antiarrhythmic drugs were introduced and approved by the Food and Drug Administration, and others are still being tested. So far no drug has been produced that is highly effective yet devoid of undesirable effects.

In patients with demonstrated life-threatening arrhythmias, more-drastic interventions are available, such as surgery. The principle behind a surgical approach to the treatment of ventricular arrhythmias is the hypothesis that most serious arrhythmias involve the reentry phenomenon: if the pathway of reentry could be identified and interrupted, further arrhythmias could be prevented. Surgical incision of areas of the endocardium (the inner layer of the heart) determined by electrophysiological studies as likely reentry pathways has eliminated serious arrhythmias in some cases. However, such operations (requiring open-heart surgery) have not been uniformly successful. The possibility that similar results could be obtained by the simpler method of introducing a cardiac catheter into the heart and producing damage (either by burning or freezing) to a critical area of abnormal conduction is now being tested.

Patients who have been resuscitated from cardiac arrest caused by documented ventricular fibrillation can now be treated by automatic defibrillators, which can recognize ventricular fibrillation and immediately apply an electric shock capable of terminating the arrhythmia. This treatment requires surgical introduction of a wire into the surface of the heart. Initial experience with automatic defibrillators has been satisfactory, though they have not proven to be without risk.

Other Arrhythmias
Heart Block and Other Bradycardias

The interruption of conducting paths connecting the atria with the ventricles produces heart block. Impulses from the atria cannot reach and activate the ventricles, which then are at the mercy of a rather weak tertiary pacemaker, located within the ventricles, which becomes responsible for the contraction of the ventricles and thus the pumping function of the heart. The rhythm of the ventricular pacemaker is slow, averaging 30 beats a minute, and it is undependable because of occasional periods of further slowing or even

interruption of its action altogether (*ventricular standstill*). Bradycardia of 30 beats a minute may be tolerated by a patient, though it
limits activity. Bradycardia at a rate less than 20 beats a minute may
produce temporary loss of consciousness, as does ventricular standstill. Complete heart block and its complications are the principal
target of electronic pacemaker therapy.

Disturbance of the upper division of the conducting system, that
located within the atria, and malfunction of the primary pacemaker
may also produce excessive slowing or stoppage of the electrical
impulses activating cardiac action. If such malfunction is not compensated for by emergency action of the lower pacemakers, the
patient may experience such symptoms as dizziness or even loss of
consciousness (sick-sinus syndrome). The fundamental difference
between malfunction of the upper and lower divisions of the conducting system is that the former slows or stops the total action of
the heart—both the atria and the ventricles—whereas the latter
does not affect the atria, which may function normally (and may
speed up normally with exercise); the ventricles, however, respond
to a slow and fixed rate initiated by the ventricular pacemaker,
which is unrelated to the rhythm of the atria.

Both varieties of the malfunction of the conducting system, manifested as excessively slow heart rate or as pauses, may occur under
certain circumstances in healthy persons. Pronounced sinus bradycardia (rates as low as the high thirties) may be present as a result of
athletic training and be a desirable adaptation. Excessive sinus
bradycardia or pauses may also represent a response to certain reflexes, such as those initiated by nausea or cough, in which case the
person may experience faintness or syncope. Drugs that slow the
heartbeat may produce symptomatic serious bradycardia. In the
absence of heart disease these types of temporary complete A-V
block do not usually develop, with one exception: some persons are
born with an abnormal conducting system (congenital complete
heart block), which may be associated with other congenital defects
or may appear as the sole abnormality. They frequently exhibit much
faster ventricular rates than those who suffer from acquired heart
block and can lead an active life, often unaware of this problem.

Complete heart block (lower-division malfunction), more often
than not, is permanent. But it may also develop as a temporary
phenomenon in the course of acute disorders, such as acute myocar-

dial infarction, or following cardiac operations, or in response to certain stimuli in patients who have lesser conduction disturbances (first- or second-degree heart block). Assessment of potential danger from temporary bradycardia or pauses due to complete heart block can usually determine whether treatment is necessary or one can safely wait for the return of normal rhythm. One of the criteria in this decision is the rate and stability of the emergency substitute pacemaker.

As mentioned, the electronic pacemaker is the principal therapeutic tool in severe bradycardias, playing either a remedial or a prophylactic role. The remedial use of the pacemaker is needed in the great majority of cases of permanent, complete heart block as well as occasionally in permanent, severe sinus bradycardia. In most other bradycardias pacemakers are implanted as a standby. Serious conduction disturbances developing in the course of acute cardiac diseases often require the temporary use of a pacemaker, in which case the pulse generator is placed outside the body.

Permanent pacemaker therapy involves two decisions—whether a pacemaker is needed and, if so, whether a single-chamber or dual-chamber unit is indicated. The single-chamber pacemaker can operate in a remedial or standby role, stimulating the atria or the ventricles; it is the less expensive of the two, simpler in design and probably longer-lasting. Dual-chamber pacemakers can sense abnormal slowing of atria or ventricles and stimulate the appropriate chamber; furthermore, they can transmit normal sinus impulses from an atrium to a blocked ventricle, preserving the normal interval between them. The most important use of the dual-chamber pacemaker is in patients with permanent complete heart block, whose atria usually respond to the normal sinus node impulses but whose ventricles beat at an independent, slow, fixed rate. Here the normal variation of the heart rate in response to exercise or excitement displayed by the atria can be transmitted to the ventricles, which with a single-chamber pacemaker would operate at a fixed rate.

Preexcitation Arrhythmias

The phenomenon of *preexcitation*, known as *Wolff-Parkinson-White syndrome*, is related to a congenital abnormality of the heart in which an accessory tract conducts impulses from the atria to the ventricles. This tract is located in a different part of the heart than the normal conduction system. It can short-circuit the conduction between the two chambers (the normal impulse is delayed within the A-V node) and stimulate prematurely certain portions of the ventricular muscle. As a result, the electrocardiogram shows a pronounced distortion of the QRS complexes, which could be mistaken for serious heart disease. Yet in most persons with this abnormality the heart is structurally and functionally normal in all other respects, and they remain unaware of the existence of this anomaly until they undergo an electrocardiogram for some unrelated reason. In a small number of such persons, however, the abnormal bypass tract is a source of disabling or even life-threatening arrhythmias. The disparity between the conduction time through the normal channels and the bypass tract may under certain circumstances cause reentry tachycardias, which permit an impulse reaching the ventricle by way of either tract to return to the atrium via the other pathway. If atrial fibrillation or flutter develops, there may be an unusually rapid ventricular rate—up to 300 beats a minute—which normally would be averted by the A-V node. Some patients can be treated medically by antiarrhythmic drugs. If no effective and safe drugs for controlling the arrhythmias can be found, catheter ablation can be performed to sever the abnormal tracts. This procedure has been found more consistently successful than other catheter ablation used in controlling intractable tachycardias. If catheter ablation fails, a surgical ablation may be used.

Chapter Seven

Cardiac Emergencies

The staff of an emergency unit sees a wide spectrum of heart problems, ranging from minor complaints by worried patients to fatal or near-fatal heart attacks. The identification of a sudden change in the state of someone's health as a problem related to the heart is usually made by the patient or a family member on the basis of symptoms such as loss of consciousness, chest pain, shortness of breath, and palpitations. Each of these can be caused by heart disease or by diseases of other organs; furthermore, they may reflect anxiety over a minor complaint.

True cardiac emergencies are usually promptly recognized by medical staff, and appropriate action is taken either in the emergency unit or on transfer to a hospital. The fatal or near-fatal emergencies include

sudden cardiac death

cardiac arrest

syncope

shock

Sudden Cardiac Death

Sudden death is usually defined as unexpected death due to natural causes, with a collapse taking place without warning or preceded by symptoms for no longer than one hour. (The World Health Organization defines sudden death in much broader terms, accepting precollapse symptoms lasting as long as 24 hours; but most physicians recognize the one-hour limit.) Instantaneous death without warning is very common; symptoms, if any, preceding loss of consciousness almost always involve chest pain or shortness of breath.

The principal causes of sudden cardiac death include ventricular fibrillation, ventricular standstill, acute failure of a ventricle, and catastrophic complication (e.g. cardiac rupture). Autopsy performed after a sudden cardiac death often fails to determine the cause of death, for ventricular fibrillation has no pathologically identifiable features. Only in a minority of cases is a clear-cut explanation of the event available, such as a thrombus in a proximal portion of a principal coronary artery, a large pulmonary embolus, or cardiac rupture. In most cases autopsy reveals general cardiac impairment, such as coronary-artery disease; occasionally the heart may be structurally normal. Coronary-artery disease is by far the commonest cause of sudden cardiac death. Other causes include aortic stenosis and hypertrophic cardiomyopathy.

Sudden cardiac death ranks high among pressing public-health problems. Close to half a million cardiac patients die suddenly each year in the United States. Most sudden cardiac deaths occur in patients with serious heart disease. Yet there is a significant group of patients in the early stages of coronary-artery disease in whom measures aimed at prevention of sudden cardiac death and at early recognition of and resuscitation from ventricular fibrillation can yield good results with a structurally normal heart.

Cardiac Arrest

When the heart suddenly ceases to pump effectively it is said to be in *cardiac arrest*. This condition is characterized by loss of consciousness resulting from the absence of blood supply to the brain. It is similar to sudden cardiac death, except that rescue efforts initiated within a few minutes of the attack can resuscitate the heart. Delayed resuscitation may reestablish the circulation but often results in "brain death"—irreversible damage to the brain, which is more sensitive to lack of oxygen than any other organ. Loss of consciousness is abrupt, and the pulses disappear. In most cases cardiac arrest is caused by ventricular fibrillation or very rapid ventricular tachycardia.

Survival of cardiac arrest depends on initiating effective treatment as soon as the mechanism of the arrest is clarified. The simplest form of treatment—only occasionally effective but worth trying—is a blow on the chest in the region of the heart, which may terminate ventricular fibrillation or restart a heart in standstill. The definitive treatment of ventricular fibrillation is electric shock to the chest, or defibrillation. If a defibrillator is not immediately available, the circulation of blood can be artificially supported for a short time by periodic chest compression along with mouth-to-mouth breathing. Injection of drugs into the heart is rarely effective.

The success of electric-shock treatment of ventricular fibrillation depends largely on the underlying state of the heart. In most cases ventricular fibrillation develops as an electrical accident in a heart still capable of resuming good function (primary ventricular fibrillation), and its termination is usually successful and complete recovery possible. The long-term prognosis is thus also related to the underlying cardiac status. Ventricular fibrillation frequently develops in a fatally damaged heart (secondary ventricular fibrillation) in which normal rhythm cannot be restored or, if restored, cannot be maintained.

Another mechanism of cardiac arrest is ventricular standstill, or extreme bradycardia (see chap. 6). It occurs in complete heart block or abnormal function of the sinus node. Such patients can be treated with an external electronic pacemaker to restart heart action and maintain it until an intracardiac pacemaker can be inserted.

Syncope

Sudden loss of consciousness (occasionally associated with convulsive seizures) followed by spontaneous resumption of brain function is called syncope. Syncope is related to cardiac arrest and may have the same cause. But syncope, a more benign emergency, not only results from problems of the heart and circulation but also can be caused by malfunction of the brain (it may coincide with epilepsy and other brain-seizure disorders). There are two principal kinds of cardiocirculatory syncope—that caused by arrhythmias and that caused by disturbances of reflex control regulating the circulation.

Arrhythmias may cause syncope when the heart rate becomes

extremely slow or extremely rapid. Bradycardia or standstill may develop in complete heart block or in sinus-node disorders. Tachycardias leading to syncope include very rapid nonsustained ventricular tachycardia (at rates approaching 300 beats a minute) or a paroxysmal form of ventricular flutter or fibrillation.

Malfunction of the reflex mechanism controlling the circulation usually involves abnormal dilation of the blood vessels, which may lower systemic blood pressure and cause abnormal pooling of the blood in peripheral blood vessels. Thus not only is the control of blood pressure impaired, but reduced return of venous blood to the heart affects the quantity of blood pumped into the circulation. Another mechanism involves abnormal stimulation of the vagus nerve, which slows the heartbeat and produces sinus pauses. Among varieties of syncope related to abnormal reflexes are

simple faint, a loss of consciousness triggered by excitement or prolonged standing in the heat

syncope triggered by certain stimuli and representing exaggerated responses to reflex stimulation, such as a cough or the passing of urine

syncope associated with certain heart diseases producing abnormalities of the reflex control of the circulation, such as aortic stenosis, hypertrophic cardiomyopathy, and pulmonary hypertension

syncope due to inhibition of the function of the sinus node by reflexes originating in the arteries of the neck (carotid sinus hypersensitivity)

syncope due to inhibition of the sinus node associated with nausea

Certain types of syncope develop so abruptly that the patient may fall to the ground without warning. Such abruptness is characteristic of syncopes caused by arrhythmias (complete heart block, ventricular tachycardia or fibrillation) or associated with aortic stenosis. Syncopes related to problems of the peripheral circulation tend to develop after some warning, which enables the patient to sit down or brace the fall before losing consciousness.

Persons who are prone to syncope, or who have experienced a syncopal attack in the past, may at times become dizzy or feel faint without losing consciousness. These episodes of incomplete syncope are known as presyncopal attacks.

The prognosis of patients who have suffered one or more syncopal attacks is difficult to establish. The mechanism and cause of syncope are often uncertain, and medical evaluation may show no abnormal findings between attacks. Only occasionally are direct clues to the cause of syncope available, such as when an attack occurs while electronic monitoring is in progress or when a witness to the attack notes an absence of pulse during the attack. Some indirect clues may be helpful in evaluating patients with syncope, such as the presence of less-serious ventricular arrhythmias or atrioventricular conduction disturbances, aortic stenosis, demonstrated hypersensitivity of carotid-sinus reflex, or a tendency to faintness when the patient rapidly stands up. Often the cause of unwitnessed attacks of syncope remains undiscovered.

When findings suggest that ventricular arrhythmia may be the basis of syncopal attacks, electrophysiological testing is commonly performed. Such tests can determine whether stimulation of the heart is capable of initiating a serious arrhythmia, in which case appropriate treatment may prevent further attacks. In the presence of persistent bradycardia or conduction disturbances the placement of a permanent pacemaker is usually indicated.

Shock

When the blood supply to vital organs is severely reduced, a person goes into *shock*. The most important manifestation of shock is abnormally low arterial pressure, which is usually caused by one or more of the following mechanisms: depressed function of the cardiac pump, faulty regulation of blood pressure, and sudden loss of blood in the body.

Shock, a variety of cardiocirculatory failure, differs in many respects from heart failure, described in chapter 5. In heart failure the arterial pressure is usually maintained at a normal or near-normal level, and blood supply to vital organs is only slightly impaired; its principal deleterious consequences are related to backing up of the blood in the lungs and systemic veins, sometimes called backward heart failure. In shock, or forward failure, the blood pressure is so low that the pumping force is inadequate to maintain the circulation in various organs. There is an obvious similarity between shock and syncope: the former is partial failure of circulatory adjustment, the latter total. Furthermore, shock represents a prolonged state, whereas syncope is of very short duration. Reduced blood supply to the brain in shock often causes extreme fatigue, restlessness, confusion, and even a semicomatose state. Reduced blood flow to the skin affects temperature control: the skin becomes cool, and a cold perspiration is common. Pallor with bluish tinge (cyanosis) may also be observed.

Shock is a persistent state with a low probability of spontaneous improvement. The prognosis of shock varies widely and depends on its cause and the response to treatment. The most common causes of shock are noncardiac; they include severe infection, serious allergic reaction (*anaphylactic shock*), serious hemorrhage, intense pain, and catastrophic events in the gastrointestinal tract, such as perforation of an organ.

The least reversible, and hence most serious, form of shock is *cardiogenic shock*, produced by a sudden reduction in the pumping efficiency of a cardiac ventricle. The commonest cause of cardiogenic shock is myocardial infarction (due either to the initial injury to the heart muscle or to a later major complication). Cardiogenic shock may also develop as a result of sudden severe overload of the heart, such as rupture of a cardiac valve or massive pulmonary embolism. A state similar to shock but not directly related to malfunction of the cardiac muscle is *pericardial tamponade*, accumulation of fluid in the sac around the heart that compresses the heart and interferes with its pumping (see chap. 10). Shock may also result from rapid ectopic tachycardia.

The prognosis of cardiogenic shock is always guarded. The mortality rate under drug therapy or insertion of an intraaortic balloon pump remains high. Elimination or amelioration of the cause of cardiogenic shock is occasionally possible by surgical means.

Other Cardiac Emergencies

Patients entering an emergency unit with chest pain, a common event, are preferentially evaluated for possible acute myocardial infarction. A diagnosis of infarction calls for immediate intervention, and the relief of pain may have to take second place to prompt diagnosis. If the cause of the pain is identified as myocardial ischemia (diminished blood supply to the heart muscle), the medical staff must consider whether the problem is reversible and temporary (angina pectoris) or the heart muscle has sustained permanent damage (myocardial infarction). This question may not be answerable in the emergency unit, in which case it is usually necessary to admit the patient to the hospital for observation and further evaluation.

Other cardiovascular conditions causing sudden onset of severe chest pain include pulmonary embolism, pericarditis, and aortic dissection. Noncardiac conditions associated with chest pain severe enough to bring a patient to an emergency unit include gastrointestinal disease (hiatus hernia, esophageal spasm) and pulmonary disease (pleurisy, pneumonia, pneumothorax). Such pain may also originate in various structures of the chest wall—nerves, muscles, or the junction between the ribs and the sternum.

As explained in this chapter, arrhythmias are responsible for the majority of cases of cardiac arrest or cardiac syncope. However, patients are often sufficiently alarmed about less-serious arrhythmias to seek emergency medical care. A common condition in this category is paroxysmal tachycardia or atrial fibrillation, which may be perceived as severe pounding of the heart, even though it may not produce any abnormality in the cardiac or circulatory function. The emergency unit must decide whether to admit the patient to the hospital or administer drugs and send the patient home. Most supraventricular tachycardias can be promptly terminated by appropriate intervention, and if no underlying heart disease is present, hospitalization is usually unnecessary. Atrial flutter or fibrillation may or may not respond to treatment in the emergency unit. If the ventricular rate is above 150 beats a minute, hospitalization is frequently advisable. Ventricular tachycardia requires prompt intervention and, because of its implications, admission to the hospital.

Chapter Eight

Atherosclerosis and Coronary-Artery Disease

Atherosclerosis is a specific disease of the *intima* (inner layer) of the arteries, not necessarily related to aging, and is responsible for the most prevalent serious disease of the heart, coronary-artery disease. It typically affects the aorta and the arteries supplying blood to the heart, the brain, and the lower extremities. It should not be confused with *arteriosclerosis*, commonly known as hardening of the arteries, a degenerative process affecting the arteries that is a part of aging. It affects the arterial intima as well as the *media* (middle layer), producing abnormalities that generally do not have adverse effects on the flow of blood in the arteries.

Atherosclerotic Coronary-Artery Disease

Atherosclerosis does not uniformly affect the arterial intima but is localized, involving small foci inside the arteries. It is only when the localized lesions become large enough to interfere with the flow of blood that atherosclerosis produces serious consequences. Coronary arteries are the most vulnerable to lesions restricting blood flow because the heart has the highest rate of using and extracting oxygen from the blood and is very sensitive to its lack. Furthermore, coronary arteries do not have significant interconnections between their branches to offer alternate routes of blood supply when obstruction develops. Atherosclerosis causes a variety of lesions inside coronary arteries; from the standpoint of heart disease, however, the most important lesion is the *atherosclerotic plaque*, a small blisterlike protrusion of the intima into the lumen (cavity) of the artery, which can produce stenosis.

The atherosclerotic plaque consists of firm fibrous tissue surrounding a softer center containing fatty substances, cholesterol crystals, and other debris. A plaque in a coronary artery does not significantly interfere with blood flow until the obstruction reaches at least 60 percent of the lumen. The development of a plaque of sufficient size to interfere with blood flow is a slow process, usually taking many years. When the plaque begins to affect blood flow, large collateral channels connecting the branches of the affected artery with those of other coronary arteries may start to develop, thereby supplying the needed blood. The normal interconnections between healthy coronary arteries are tiny branches capable of supplying only minute quantities of blood to the occluded artery in an emergency. However, the gradual progression of coronary stenosis stimulates growth of these collateral interconnections, which often become large enough to take over the entire blood supply from a completely occluded artery. Thus nature may provide a bypass to a stenosed or occluded coronary artery.

The most serious consequences of coronary atherosclerosis are produced by certain complications of this process. These are

rupture of a plaque

hemorrhage into the wall of an artery

formation of a thrombus inside an artery

Each of these complications increases abruptly the degree of stenosis, which usually results in a significant progression of symptoms and other consequences of coronary disease.

In rupture of a plaque (referred to as a "coronary accident"), much as in rupture of an abscess, the fibrous covering splits, permitting its soft contents to spill into the artery. In response, white blood cells and platelets immediately aggregate at the point of rupture to repair the damage. This process not only increases the stenosis but may also stimulate the formation of a thrombus, which could further reduce the lumen of the affected artery or close it off completely. The effect of this kind of accident on the heart depends on how much increase in stenosis has taken place and on whether compensatory collateral arteries are available. Hemorrhage into the arterial wall (*subintimal hemorrhage*) can also suddenly increase the degree of stenosis, although its effects are seldom as dramatic as those of rupture of a plaque. Thrombus formation inside a coronary artery, though a common sequel to plaque rupture, may also occur without it, stimulated by an area of damage in the intima. Coronary thrombosis is the principal cause of myocardial infarction.

The cause of atherosclerosis is not definitely known. Among theories dealing with the initiation of the atherosclerotic process the most widely accepted is the injury hypothesis, which suggests that a localized injury to the intima of a coronary artery is the point of origin of atherosclerotic lesions. It is well recognized that the early stages of atherosclerosis may develop even in adolescents and children. Yellow fatty streaks, the visible precursors of atherosclerotic plaques, are frequently found in arteries of healthy young adults. Local injury to the intima may attract fatty substances, which are then deposited there, initiating a rather complex process leading eventually to large, clinically significant plaques.

Atherosclerotic coronary-artery disease is not distributed evenly around the globe. Its incidence in the developing nations is much lower than in developed countries; in some tribes of Africa it is virtually nonexistent. A major reason for this difference is the amount and type of fatty substances in the diet. Diets rich in foods containing saturated fatty acids and cholesterol, such as prevail in most Western nations, enhance the development of coronary disease.

The principal building block of atherosclerotic plaques is cholesterol—a ubiquitous substance, important in all cell structures, which in combination with proteins is transported in the bloodstream as *lipoprotein*. Among the various types of lipoproteins two play important roles in the development of coronary atherosclerosis: *low-density lipoproteins* (LDLs), which transport most of the cholesterol and tend to deposit it in arterial lesions, and *high-density lipoproteins* (HDLs), which are capable of removing cholesterol from injured arterial walls and transporting it to the liver for use in forming bile.

The relationship between the amount of cholesterol circulating in the blood (serum cholesterol) and coronary-artery disease is well documented, and the level of serum cholesterol is used as a predictor of coronary disease. That level in the Western population ranges between 150 and 300 mg per 100 milliliters of serum (mg percent). Serum cholesterol is greatly influenced by the amount of saturated fat and cholesterol in the ingested food, although the varying ability of persons to metabolize fatty substances plays an important role as well. The present view is that a desirable level of serum cholesterol in adults is less than 200 mg percent, and a level above 240 mg percent is too high and may require intervention to reduce it. Whereas total serum cholesterol is the widely used risk factor, it is now generally accepted that LDLs ("bad cholesterol") are implicated in atherosclerotic plaque formation, whereas the HDLs ("good cholesterol") inhibit plaque formation. Higher ranges of serum cholesterol may reflect a high-fat diet or inefficient fat metabolism. In one disease, *familial hyperlipidemia* (it is usually hereditary), grossly abnormal metabolism of fatty substances may raise serum cholesterol as high as 1000 mg percent. There are several varieties of this metabolic disorder, most of which are associated with premature and severe coronary-artery disease.

Triglycerides, another group of chemical substances transported with lipoproteins, are also considered predictors of coronary-artery disease if serum levels are abnormally high, although this relationship is not as clear as that involving LDL cholesterol.

The atherosclerotic process affects men more often than it affects women. It is thought to be stimulated or retarded by the presence or absence of certain risk factors. Inasmuch as the relationship between risk factors and coronary-artery disease is based on statistics rather than direct observation, the importance of these risk factors is not always clear-cut and is the subject of controversy. Risk factors that can be influenced by therapy are of particular importance since their reduction may arrest the progress of atherosclerosis or even cause its regression. Others merely identify subjects at higher-than-average risk of heart attacks.

The three risk factors accepted by most experts as central to address in preventive treatment of atherosclerosis are hypercholesterolemia (high serum cholesterol), smoking, and hypertension (high blood pressure). Risk factors whose role is less established or is questionable include stress, obesity, sedentary habits, diabetes, and the so-called coronary-prone personality. Risk factors that cannot be altered by treatment include male sex and a family history of heart attacks early in life.

Risk factors for coronary-artery disease should be addressed whenever possible by prophylactic treatment. The most aggressive and widely accepted treatment is aimed at reducing serum cholesterol. It includes two strategies—primary prevention, directed at the entire population of a given area, and secondary prevention, directed at patients who have had heart attacks or have shown other manifestations of the disease.

Primary prevention involves modifying one's diet. Since dietary restrictions may affect quality of life, primary prevention of coronary-artery disease focuses on the least disruptive adjustments in dietary habits. A healthy diet for children and adolescents, if followed by a large segment of that population, could have a significant impact on the future prevalence of coronary-artery disease. Stronger measures, such as drug therapy, are generally indicated only in persons with significant hypercholesterolemia.

Secondary prevention requires a more aggressive approach, including a stricter diet and, if indicated, drug therapy. Two classes of drugs reduce serum cholesterol—those affecting fat metabolism in the body and those interfering with fat absorption in the bowel. The latter drugs may cause gastrointestinal upset but are otherwise well tolerated and are considered safe for long-term, often lifelong, use. Powerful drugs affecting fat metabolism have now been accepted for general use, but not enough time has elapsed to determine whether long-term use of these effective drugs carries any risk to vital organs. They therefore are administered mainly when dietary means fail and the level of serum cholesterol is unusually high.

Complementing these preventive treatments of coronary-artery disease are agents that reduce the risk of thrombus formation. Evidence suggesting that small doses of aspirin may inhibit blood platelets from contributing to thrombus formation has provided a simple and inexpensive means of influencing the process that leads to heart attacks. However, the practical value of aspirin in preventing heart attacks has yet to be clearly established.

Risk modification concerning high blood pressure and smoking is treated as a general health measure rather than as a specific preventive measure in coronary-artery disease. Hypertension requires treatment irrespective of its role in coronary-artery disease; similarly, the noxious effect of tobacco, the subject of intensive antismoking campaigns, involves other diseases than atherosclerosis. The question whether risk modification can actually produce regression of existing atherosclerotic lesions has not yet been answered, though some studies suggest it can.

Sequelae of Coronary Atherosclerosis

Coronary-artery disease is related to a single consequence of atherosclerotic reduction of coronary blood flow—ischemia of the heart muscle. Myocardial ischemia is a decreased delivery of oxygen to heart muscle cells such that myocardial oxygen demand exceeds the supply of oxygen through the coronary circulation. Thus ischemia may develop if myocardial oxygen requirements increase but supply remains the same or if such requirements remain stable but blood flow supplying oxygen is reduced. Increased myocardial oxygen demand is related to cardiac workload. For example, exercise steeply increases the oxygen requirements of the heart muscle; a similar effect, though less pronounced, is produced by factors elevating arterial pressure.

To explain the relationship between oxygen supply and demand, we need to understand the concept of *coronary reserve*. Approximately 20 percent of the maximum capacity of the coronary arteries to supply the heart muscle with oxygen is required by a person at rest. The remaining 80 percent of potential blood flow represents the coronary reserve available to take care of increased cardiac oxygen demands. An atherosclerotic plaque may grow to the point where coronary blood flow is affected, reducing the coronary reserve from 80 percent to 60 percent. In this case myocardial ischemia would develop only when the full reserve was required, such as during strenuous exercise, at which time the person would experience chest pain. Further growth of a plaque eliminates more cardiac reserve, producing chest pain with less-strenuous activity. More-severe stenosis may reduce coronary reserve to the point where relatively light activity produces ischemia. Myocardial ischemia (and its accompanying chest pain) may also result from other factors raising myocardial oxygen demands, such as increases in blood pressure or heart rate due to stress or excitement. Ischemia caused by increased myocardial oxygen demands is by definition reversible, for adequate oxygen supply resumes as soon as oxygen requirements return to normal (basal) levels.

Myocardial ischemia caused by reduced blood supply without any increase in myocardial oxygen demand may be temporary. A spasm of a coronary artery may restrict normal blood flow through it, and normal myocardial function returns once the spasm is relieved. More serious is a permanent injury to the myocardium, which may develop if ischemia persists for at least 15 to 20 minutes (according to present estimates). The ultimate variety of reduced blood and oxygen supply to the myocardium is permanent occlusion of a coronary artery by a thrombus, resulting in myocardial infarction.

Myocardial ischemia can have several effects on the heart—faulty contraction of the affected portion of the heart muscle (reduced or absent contractions); left ventricular failure, if the ischemia affects a large area of the myocardium; and, occasionally, ventricular arrhythmias. The consequences of temporary ischemia disappear either spontaneously or in response to interventions (such as taking nitroglycerin), provided adequate blood supply is restored within the critical time limit.

Ischemia can be detected by means of the following diagnostic findings:

electrocardiographic changes consisting of a temporary shift of the S-T segment (fig. 27)

reversible abnormalities of isotopic perfusion scans performed in connection with stress tests (fig. 16, p. 39)

reversible abnormalities of left ventricular wall motion

Electrocardiographic abnormalities characteristic of ischemia may show up over the course of a Holter monitor test or during a treadmill exercise test. They may also appear when monitoring hospitalized patients during a spontaneous attack of chest pain.

In the treadmill stress test the workload on the heart is gradually increased by speeding up the treadmill and adding a slight incline. The goal of the test is to attain 90 percent of the predicted maximal heart rate during exercise for the person being tested (ranging between 120 and 150 beats a minute). A multilead electrocardiogram records during the test; the patient is also monitored for

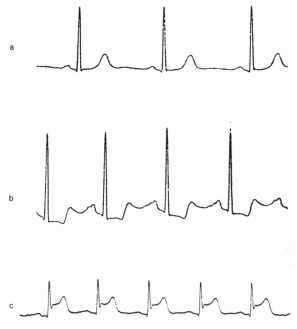

Figure 27. Single electrocardiographic leads
exemplifying changes produced by myocardial
ischemia. (a) Normal configuration. (b) Complexes showing depressed S-T segments,
signifying moderate myocardial ischemia (e.g.
during treadmill exercise test), which return to
normal when the normal flow is restored.
(c) Complexes showing elevated S-T segments
signifying severe ischemia (myocardial injury),
such as seen during early stages of myocardial
infarction.

changes in blood pressure and the development of chest pain. In
the presence of ischemia the S-T segment of the electrocardiogram
shifts downward or, if ischemia is unusually severe, upward. Information concerning the severity of ischemia can be obtained from
the extent of the S-T segment shifts, the amount of exercise required to provoke ischemia, and the time needed for the S-T segment to resume a normal position after the test.

A Holter monitor test may reveal ischemia in the development
of S-T segment depression during daily activities. Special equipment sensitive to S-T segment changes must be employed (the

primary objective of the Holter monitor test is the detection of arrhythmias). Spontaneous attacks of angina in hospitalized patients provide an additional opportunity to detect ischemia (or support its diagnosis) by observing temporary S-T segment shifts in the electrocardiogram during the attack of chest pain.

The diagnosis of ischemia by means of electrocardiographic abnormalities does have limitations. This method is most reliable when the control electrocardiogram (taken when the patient is at rest) is normal. Certain abnormalities in the control electrocardiogram may reduce the reliability of a test or even make a conclusive diagnosis of ischemia impossible.

The diagnostic use of isotopic scanning tests has been described in chapter 3. The test is performed in conjunction with the treadmill or pharmacological stress test and complements its findings. Whereas some indication of the severity of ischemia can be obtained from electrocardiographic changes, isotopic scanning can reveal the amount of heart muscle affected by the ischemia. Isotopic scan is of particular importance in cases where the electrocardiographic test is inconclusive or is incapable of supplying diagnostic information because of preexisting distortion of the complexes.

Under ordinary circumstances the electrocardiographic treadmill stress test is the principal means of diagnosing ischemia. Other procedures, such as the isotopic perfusion test and nuclide ventriculogram, steeply increase the cost of the diagnosis and are carried out only if specifically indicated.

Once ischemia has been diagnosed, further evaluation of the extent of coronary-artery disease is often made by means of coronary angiography (see chap. 3). The film taken after injecting the contrast material into the coronary arteries shows the distribution of blood through each coronary-artery system and displays any stenosis and occlusion of the branches (fig. 28). Angiography can also reveal collateral connections between arterial branches. This test is essential for determining the precise location of atherosclerotic plaques and evaluating the extent of coronary-artery disease. It is a prerequisite to such interventions as coronary angioplasty or bypass surgery. It should be emphasized, however, that tests for ischemia and angiography complement each other: angiography shows the lesion that may be responsible for ischemia but does not prove the presence of ischemia.

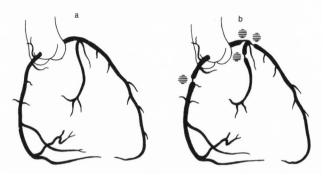

Figure 28. Coronary arteriograms (in actuality only one artery is visualized at a time). (a) Normal coronary arteriogram. (b) Coronary arteriogram showing four areas of severe stenosis (indicated by shaded circles). (Reprinted, by permission, from Arthur Selzer, *Principles and Practice of Clinical Cardiology* [Philadelphia: W. B. Saunders, 1983]).

Features of Coronary-Artery Disease and Its Course

Myocardial ischemia is the common denominator for all manifestations of coronary-artery disease. Thus a disease responsible for more deaths than any other condition is the result of a single mechanism caused by lesions obstructing the coronary arteries. Interestingly, there is no general agreement on one term to describe the effect of ischemia on the heart. The logical and most appropriate term to incorporate all consequences of ischemia, "ischemic heart disease," has not been widely accepted and is only occasionally used. Less precise terms such as "arteriosclerotic heart disease," "coronary-artery disease," "coronary heart disease," or simply "coronary disease" are predominantly used in medical writings and parlance. Its course and outcome depend entirely on how large a portion of the heart muscle is deprived of oxygen and for how long. Coronary-artery disease occurs in the form of specific syndromes categorized according to their features, prognosis, and need for intervention. In a sense they represent stages of the disease, though the patient does not necessarily progress steadily from milder to more serious syndromes.

Manifestations of coronary-artery disease fall into two categories—(1) acute short-term illness or (2) a chronic state with continuous or intermittent symptoms. Chronic coronary syndromes include

asymptomatic coronary disease (including silent ischemia)

stable angina pectoris

chronic pump failure

The acute coronary syndromes are

sudden coronary death

acute myocardial infarction

unstable angina pectoris

Since pump failure is the final stage of coronary-artery disease and usually follows myocardial infarction, it will be discussed last in this chapter.

Asymptomatic Coronary Disease

Atherosclerotic plaques have to reach considerable size before producing myocardial ischemia, which usually causes patients to experience chest pain (angina pectoris). Because of the prevalence of coronary-artery disease in the West and the slow growth of most atherosclerotic plaques, some coronary-artery disease can be found in a large segment of the population, as shown by autopsies of healthy persons who died a violent death (such as were performed on the bodies of young soldiers killed in the Korean War). Thus symptom-producing coronary-artery disease represents only a fraction of the incidence of such disease in the general population.

In asymptomatic coronary-artery disease atherosclerotic plaques have not reached the critical size to interfere with coronary blood flow. However, in a subgroup of persons with asymptomatic coronary-artery disease, ischemia is induced much as in stable angina pectoris, but no chest pain results. This phenomenon, commonly known as silent ischemia, can be detected by conventional diagnostic methods, such as the treadmill exercise test, isotopic perfusion test, and Holter monitor test. The reason why myocardial ischemia in some instances fails to be signaled by chest pain has not been adequately determined. Many patients with stable angina pectoris suffer from attacks of silent ischemia in addition to attacks of chest pain; that is, myocardial ischemia occurs more frequently than they are aware of.

The discovery of silent ischemia in otherwise healthy persons, usually during a routine checkup, presents a dilemma. It is not yet known whether the prognosis of such patients is worse than that of similar people who do not show ischemia. It is uncertain whether the performance of invasive (angiographic) studies in cases of silent ischemia is indicated and whether intervention other than primary prevention of atherosclerosis is advisable.

Stable Angina Pectoris

Angina pectoris is the classical earmark of coronary-artery disease. Stable angina pectoris, a chronic state, can persist unchanged for years. It indicates that a patient with reduced coronary reserve has no symptoms at rest, but during exercise or activities the amount of oxygen supplied to the heart by the coronary circulation may become insufficient to cover the increased demands. The threshold for provoking chest pain may be constant (that is, the same amount of exercise may always produce pain), but often the appearance of chest pain is contingent on an additional factor, such as walking in cold weather or having eaten a heavy meal. Some patients develop angina in response to excitement or anger. Since in stable angina pectoris a provoking factor is responsible for chest pain, a careful analysis of the circumstances leading up to the appearance of pain is vital. For example, an attack of chest pain at night may prove to have followed a nightmare and thus have been provoked. By contrast, unprovoked nocturnal pain is a sign of unstable angina.

Chest pain in stable angina subsides with rest or disappears promptly when the patient takes sublingually a tablet of nitroglycerin. The effect of stable angina on the life-style of patients varies greatly. Mild angina may be controlled without medication by eliminating strenuous exercise. When anginal attacks begin to interfere with ordinary activities, medical treatment may be able to alleviate the symptoms. Gradual changes in stable angina occur in both directions: chest pain may develop during less-strenuous activities than in the past or may only be provoked by more-strenuous exercise than previously. Occasionally angina may disappear altogether.

An apparent worsening of symptoms is best explained by slow progression of atherosclerotic disease, and seeming improvement by development of effective coronary collaterals. Only when acceleration of angina occurs abruptly should the diagnosis of unstable angina be made.

Prognosis of stable angina pectoris is in principle favorable. Statistical studies of large numbers of patients have shown that those with stable angina who have not sustained ischemic damage to the heart muscle (caused by myocardial infarction or a lesser coronary syndrome) have a life expectancy only slightly lower than that of others their age in the general population. In some patients the benign course is interrupted by one of the more dangerous acute syndromes, but they are obviously in the minority. For purposes of prognosis it is customary to subdivide patients with stable angina into those whose coronary angiogram shows significant disease in only one coronary artery, those with "two-vessel disease," and those with "three-vessel disease." However, statistical differences in life expectancy among these three groups is rather small so long as the left ventricle remains healthy.

Evaluating stable angina pectoris requires a general survey of the cardiac status. The possibility that noncoronary ischemia (such as results from aortic stenosis or hypertrophic cardiomyopathy) may be responsible for the symptoms has to be considered. The performance of the heart must be reviewed to determine whether it has suffered myocardial damage. After the presence of ischemia has been confirmed by a treadmill stress test or other diagnostic procedures, many physicians arrange for coronary angiography, though others omit invasive tests if the patient promptly and satisfactorily responds to medical treatment.

Treatment of stable angina involves one of two approaches—medical therapy or interventional therapy (including coronary angioplasty and coronary bypass surgery). Medical therapy of stable angina pectoris is based primarily on the ability of nitroglycerin to provide rapid relief from chest pain. This drug is effective in the form of small tablets that dissolve when placed by the patient under the tongue, once the sole method to control anginal attacks. The 1970s and 1980s saw the introduction of some other effective drugs for preventing attacks of angina. Their use has revolutionized medical therapy of angina pectoris. They are beta-adrenergic blocking agents, calcium channel blocking agents, and long-acting nitrates having nitroglycerinlike effect. In addition, nitroglycerin can now be administered in slow-release form, as tablets or ointment in patches placed on the skin.

Interventional therapy is effective in controlling angina and is used widely. There is no consensus, however, regarding its indications. The most widely accepted, conservative criteria for intervention include the following:

stenosis of the left main coronary artery

failure to respond to medical therapy

the presence of coronary lesions shown by angiography to be precarious (such as proximal stenosis of the left anterior coronary branch)

evidence that ischemia involves large sections of cardiac muscle

Coronary angioplasty was developed in 1978 and has been a popular alternative to bypass surgery (see fig. 19, p. 55). The technique of coronary angioplasty is described in chapter 4. Originally conceived as a method of dilating proximal stenosis of one of the three major coronary branches in single-vessel disease, the use of this procedure has now been extended to handling lesions in smaller coronary branches and in two- or three-vessel disease.

Angioplasty has proven immensely successful in eliminating or reducing stenosis of coronary arteries by compressing atherosclerotic plaques. However, in about 5 percent of cases the procedure can damage the arterial wall and close off the affected artery altogether. In such cases an immediate bypass operation may have to be performed: standby surgical facilities should be available in hospitals routinely performing angioplasty. Another possible complication of angioplasty is recurrence of stenosis within weeks after the procedure, which develops in 20–30 percent of cases. Repeat angioplasty is usually performed, and the probability of recurrent restenosis is greatly reduced. The advantages of angioplasty over bypass surgery are obvious: it is the simpler of the two procedures, its cost is lower, and recovery is swift.

Coronary bypass surgery provides an artificial channel connecting the aorta with the coronary artery beyond the area of stenosis or occlusion (see figs. 29 and 30). The operation is performed under

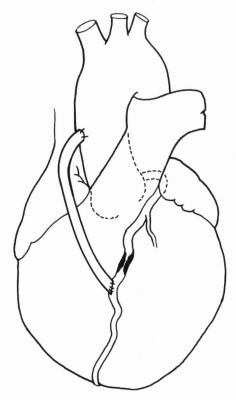

Figure 29. Coronary bypass graft. A portion of a
saphenous vein from the patient's leg is used to
connect the ascending aorta with a coronary
branch beyond the point of severe stenosis.

direct vision as open-heart surgery: a segment of a saphenous vein
(a superficial vein running under the skin of the inner surface of a
leg) is excised and then grafted to serve as a connecting tube between the aorta and the coronary artery. An alternate method is to
connect the lower end of the mammary artery (an artery running
inside the chest on either side of the breastbone) with the ob-
structed coronary artery.

Coronary-bypass surgery is now the most frequently performed
cardiovascular operation. More than three hundred thousand of
these procedures are performed in the United States annually. The
risk of the operation is relatively small, with mortality rates of 1–5
percent in hospitals with experienced cardiac surgical terms. Pa-

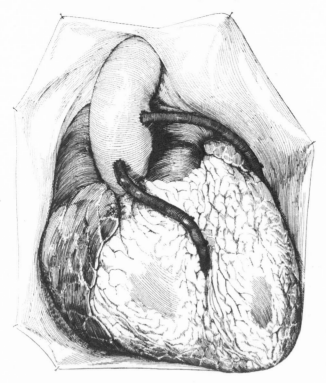

Figure 30. Coronary bypass graft as seen with the chest open.

tients generally tolerate the operation well, and results are usually satisfactory, although closure of the bypass graft occurs in a significant number of cases, particularly if the graft is connected to a smaller coronary branch.

Interventional treatment of stable angina as well as coronary-artery disease does not represent a cure. Apart from unsuccessful results of the intervention (restenosis after angioplasty, graft closure after an operation) progression of the disease in other coronary branches may bring about new symptoms or more-serious manifestations of coronary-artery disease. Repeat operations or angioplasties are often needed even if the original procedure is fully successful. Yet interventional treatment may delay the progression of the disease by years or even decades. Furthermore, enhanced quality of life and freedom from symptoms as a result of interventional therapy have made it an exciting advance in the management of heart disease. However, statistical proof that patients who have undergone interventional treatment live longer than those treated medically is not yet available, except in some special high-risk situations. This lack of proof is in part related to the fact that the prognosis of patients with stable angina pectoris who have never suffered a myocardial infarction and have normal function in the left ventricle is good.

Unstable Angina Pectoris

Inherent in the concept of stable angina pectoris is the principle that myocardial ischemia is caused by increased cardiac demand for oxygen. Attacks of chest pain are predictable since each attack has a definable cause, such as exercise or excitement. This predictability is missing in attacks of unstable angina, where oxygen supply to the heart muscle fluctuates irrespective of myocardial oxygen demands.

Unstable angina pectoris, in the broadest sense of the term, includes many situations in which chest pain does not follow a chronic, repetitive pattern. It occupies an intermediate position between stable angina and myocardial infarction and is classified as an acute coronary syndrome. As such, we can distinguish the following patterns:

rapid increase in frequency and severity of attacks of angina pectoris ("crescendo angina")

onset of angina provoked by a low level of activity

a combination of exercise-induced attacks of angina and unprovoked attacks at rest

occasional recurrent attacks of angina at night

a high concentration of unprovoked anginal attacks at rest (usually several attacks a day)

prolonged attacks of angina at rest (15 minutes or longer)

Current medical opinion places the cause of unstable angina close to that of myocardial infarction, namely an acute change inside a major coronary artery, most commonly rupture of an atherosclerotic plaque. Though the course of unstable angina is unpredictable, the six patterns are listed here in order from least to most precarious. All cases of unstable angina should be considered for intensive hospital treatment, which is mandatory in the more serious varieties. Prolonged attacks of chest pain at rest are usually handled as suspected myocardial infarctions. Since the difference between unstable angina and myocardial infarction depends on the reversibility of ischemia, sometimes the two can be distinguished only after noting a series of changes in electrocardiographic readings and cardiac enzymes. Rapidly recurring attacks of angina at rest that are of shorter duration often are precursors of myocardial infarction. In some patients suffering occasional recurrent attacks of nocturnal angina, unstable angina may be caused by periodic spasm of a coronary artery (analogous to attacks of migraine caused by spasm of cerebral arteries). Coronary-artery spasms have distinctive features. An electrocardiogram taken during such an attack shows an elevated S-T segment instead of the depressed one typical of ischemia at rest. This angina, called variant angina or Prinzmetal's angina, displays electrocardiographic patterns identical with the early changes of myocardial infarction, but the patterns return to normal promptly after the attack. Many such patients have only a minor degree of coronary-artery disease; sometimes in fact the coronary arteries are entirely normal. The prognosis for such patients is much more favorable than for those with other varieties of unstable angina, and their response to medical treatment is usually excellent; in these cases intervention therapy does not help and is contraindicated.

Management of unstable angina is aimed at prompt control of symptoms for patients both in the hospital and at home. Hospitalized patients usually require continuous intravenous administration of drugs. In addition to antianginal drugs, anticoagulants (to prevent clot formation) and thrombolytics (to dissolve clots) may be used. Interventional therapy is often considered, requiring coronary angiograms. Both angiography and interventional treatment may have to be performed as emergency procedures if symptoms cannot be controlled by medical therapy.

As an acute coronary syndrome, unstable angina has an unpredictable outcome: it may progress to myocardial infarction, it may settle into stable angina, or it may cease altogether or change into stable angina. If interventional therapy is performed, either angioplasty or bypass operation may restore the patient to an asymptomatic state.

Acute Myocardial Infarction

Myocardial infarction—a heart attack, in common parlance—affects at least three-quarters of a million Americans a year. It is an acute event in the course of atherosclerotic coronary-artery disease; after the initial attack of chest pain it takes approximately six weeks for the body to repair the damage to the heart muscle by forming a firm scar. Present standards of care require that the early treatment be administered in the intensive-care unit of a hospital (or in a coronary-care unit if available), followed by further care at a routine hospital facility. The average hospital stay is one week, with wide variations depending on the type of myocardial infarction and the possibility of complications.

The term "infarction" means damage to a tissue in the body caused by depriving it of blood supply. Myocardial infarction results from myocardial ischemia that has lasted too long for the affected tissue to recover and has become irreversible, thereby producing necrosis (death associated with softening) of a portion of the heart muscle. Myocardial infarction is almost always caused by an intracoronary accident (described earlier in this chapter) and in most cases involves formation of a intracoronary thrombus occluding the coronary artery at the point of the accident (usually rupture of a plaque). The size of the infarction—in other words, the extent of the damage to the myocardium—depends on the size of the occluded coronary artery, the location of the occlusion, and the availability of protective collateral circulation. If irreversible ischemia affects a large portion of the muscle of the left ventricle, the patient may not survive; hence the first few hours after the initial chest pain are critical, and mortality in that period is high. However, ventricular fibrillation leading to cardiac arrest may also develop in patients with smaller infarctions; they can be successfully resuscitated and may completely recover.

The outlook for patients suffering a myocardial infarction who reach the hospital alive is favorable. Two studies dealing with early treatment, based on some 26,000 cases, showed that the survival rate for patients admitted to a hospital with myocardial infarction is greater than 87 percent when they are treated conventionally and 90 percent when thrombolytic drugs are administered.

Diagnosis of Myocardial Infarction. A patient's description of an attack of chest pain and associated symptoms is often a sufficient basis for suspecting acute myocardial infarction. Further medical evaluation in the emergency unit, or later in the hospital, may confirm the diagnosis. Myocardial infarction can be classified by its size and location. The most extensive infarction is a *transmural infarction,* involving all layers of the wall of the left ventricle. It is also referred to as a Q-wave infarction because of certain electrocardiographic abnormalities. It can affect the front wall of the ventricle (anterior infarction) or the lower back wall (inferior infarction). This type of infarction causes the most serious damage and leads to the most complications. *Subendocardial infarction* affects the inner layer of the left ventricular muscle. Infarction of the right ventricle is less common than that of the left ventricle and as a rule represents an extension of an inferior infarction of the left ventricle. Myocardial infarction may also be less well defined, involving smaller sections of the myocardium, sometimes in more than one area. Furthermore, there are instances in which myocardial infarction can only be suspected, not proven.

The characteristic feature of the initial attack of myocardial infarction is chest pain, usually in the center of the chest behind the breastbone or across the upper portion of the front of the chest. Pain may radiate to one or both arms and the neck. The severity of the pain varies, but it develops without provocation and persists, usually unrelieved by nitroglycerin. About one-half of patients having their first myocardial infarction experience chest pain for the first time during that attack. In others it may be preceded by stable or unstable angina pectoris of varying duration. Other symptoms may accompany or follow the attack of chest pain—dyspnea, nausea with or without vomiting, pallor with cold perspiration, faintness or dizziness, and collapse.

Classic attacks of myocardial infarction are usually easy to identify, not only for a physician but also for the person stricken. There are many instances, however, when an attack may prove difficult to diagnose. Chest pain may be in unusual locations or so slight as to be dismissed by the patient. Occasionally pain is altogether absent;

in that case the patient may merely experience shortness of breath and sudden weakness or may collapse without warning. The reaction of someone experiencing a myocardial infarction runs from shock and alarm at recognizing the onset of a serious illness to dismissal of the pain as indigestion.

The course and outcome of acute myocardial infarction relates to many factors, the most important of which is the size of the infarct. Irreversible damage to a large portion of the left ventricle, the main pumping chamber, may be incompatible with survival. If the damage involves 40 percent or more of the left ventricular musculature, the outcome is invariably fatal: cardiac arrest soon follows, and efforts to resuscitate, even when immediate, are unsuccessful. Myocardial infarcts involving less than 40 percent of the muscle vary in their effect on the cardiac function according to the size and location of the infarct (those affecting the anterior wall are most serious); possible underlying heart disease, such as damage to the heart from hypertension or previous coronary episodes; the general condition of the patient and the presence of other diseases, such as diabetes, kidney disease, or lung disease; the presence of disease in other coronary arteries than the one occluded; and the development of complications.

The relationship between the size of the infarction and the effect on cardiac function, as modified by the various secondary influences, can be presented (in an admittedly oversimplified manner) as follows:

massive myocardial infarction→sudden death

very large infarction→cardiogenic shock

large infarction→left ventricular failure

small to medium infarction→no impairment of functions

This relationship describes the initial response of the heart to the sudden damaging effect of ischemia. The overall course is further determined by the secondary sequelae of the infarction and its possible complications. Yet the initial response to the attack is critical: about one-third of all deaths resulting from myocardial infarction occur immediately after the onset or within a few hours, often before the patient reaches a hospital. Out-of-hospital resuscitation of patients can save only those with modest damage to the myocardium, that is, who have developed primary ventricular fibrillation.

Myocardial infarction produces a variety of secondary effects or complications. They most commonly develop within 48 hours of the attack and may or may not respond favorably to treatment. It should be reiterated, however, that close to 90 percent of patients admitted to the hospital survive the attack. Most enter the hospital after chest pain and associated symptoms have subsided and may feel well throughout the hospital stay. Yet their prognosis may be affected by one or more of the immediate sequelae:

Cardiogenic shock. This may develop with the initial attack, may come on gradually, or may strike suddenly later. Shock developing after a day or two of improvement is usually caused by a major complication of the infarction. Cardiogenic shock is associated with high mortality.

Arrhythmias. Ventricular arrhythmias are very common and are usually inconsequential if limited to premature beats. Monitoring of cardiac rhythm permits immediate intervention if more-serious ventricular arrhythmias develop. Atrial arrhythmias are less common and as a rule respond well to treatment.

Heart failure. This may be present at admission to the hospital or may develop later. Left ventricular failure requires immediate therapy but usually can be contained. Unresponsive heart failure, particularly if affecting both ventricles, is an unfavorable sign and often signifies an extension of the infarction to the right ventricle.

Hypotension. The patient's blood pressure is usually lower than normal following a heart attack; however, in some patients blood pressure falls below an acceptable level (but not low enough to cause shock). Appropriate treatment can rectify the problem.

Major complications of myocardial infarction include the following:

Extension of myocardial infarction. Occasionally a new attack of chest pain develops after one or two days without pain. New electrocardiographic abnormalities may show that the infarct has increased in size.

Angina pectoris. The patient may continue having attacks of chest pain after the initial attack has subsided, sometimes indicating disease in the nonoccluded branches.

Rupture of the heart. A transmural infarction may soften the infarcted muscle to the point that an opening develops connecting the ventricular chamber with the pericardial space. This complication is usually fatal, although in rare instances immediate surgery may save the patient's life.

Rupture of the ventricular septum. If the softened portion of the cardiac muscle affects the septum rather than the outside wall of the left ventricle, an opening between the left and right ventricles develops. In consequence, blood is shunted from the high-pressure left ventricle to the low-pressure right ventricle, greatly increasing the workload of the heart. Depending on the size of the opening, the result may be death, cardiogenic shock, or mild-to-moderate heart failure. Usually there is time to arrange for corrective surgery in more-serious cases. In milder cases surgery may be deferred until after recovery from the myocardial infarction.

Acute mitral regurgitation. Myocardial infarction occasionally damages one of the two papillary muscles in the left ventricle anchoring the mitral valve through the attached chordae. Such damage may produce incompetence of the mitral valve, leading to an overloading of the circulation. The effects of this complication are similar to those of rupture of the ventricular septum, and emergency surgery is often required.

Emboli in the systemic circulation. During the early stages of myocardial infarction clots may develop inside the left ventricle at the point where infarction may have damaged the endocardium. Portions of thrombi may detach themselves from the wall of the ventricle and travel in the bloodstream, producing emboli, which in turn may lead to stroke.

Pericarditis. Inflammation of the pericardium sometimes develops in the course of myocardial infarction. It is usually a benign complication and does not influence the course of the attack.

Heart block. Damage to the conducting system of the heart often produces varying degrees of conduction disturbance. This may be a transient phenomenon requiring no intervention. Often, however, insertion of an electronic pacemaker is needed, either temporarily or permanently.

The diagnosis of myocardial infarction is based on three component findings—the initial attack of chest pain, a sequence of electrocardiographic changes, and the results of a blood test to determine the level of serum enzymes. The initial diagnostic evaluation is usually performed in an emergency unit. Great weight has to be placed on the patient's description of the attack since the physician's examination often contributes little to the diagnosis. The initial electrocardiogram may establish a tentative diagnosis of myocardial infarction, but full confirmation depends on two or more serially performed tests. Early testing for cardiac enzymes in the blood serum cannot contribute to the diagnosis because the characteristic rise in enzymes occurs several hours after the attack (peaking 12 to 24 hours later). Diagnostic difficulty may arise if the attack is atypical and the electrocardiographic changes are noncharacteristic or delayed. Since early treatment in an intensive-care unit is essential, patients suspected of suffering myocardial infarction are usually admitted to a hospital facility. The subsequent evaluation of doubtful cases, usually completed within 24 to 48 hours of hospitalization, can distinguish those patients whose chest pain is caused by abnormalities other than those of the heart or who are experiencing severe unstable angina without damage to the heart muscle.

The establishment of a diagnosis of myocardial infarction is only the first step in the diagnostic assessment of the problem. It is necessary to evaluate the damage to the heart and its consequences for the circulation and to recognize, or even anticipate, any change so as to provide appropriate treatment. The patient's heart rate and rhythm are continuously displayed on the cardiac monitor, the blood pressure is frequently checked, and a physical examination is performed periodically. In patients who are medically stable and feel well, observation and routine care may be all that is required. But further diagnostic procedures are available if indicated. A chest X-ray may show the presence of left ventricular failure. Echocardiographic examination or nuclide ventriculography permits an evaluation of the function of the damaged left ventricle, can provide information regarding the size and location of dead muscle tissue, and can detect clots in the left ventricle. More elaborate tests may be needed if the patient's recovery is·marred by continuing or delayed circulatory problems. Overt heart failure or shock may call for continuous monitoring of cardiac dynamics by means of a flow-directed cardiac catheter. A complete cardiac catheterization and angiographic study may become necessary if a more severe complication is suspected.

Management of Myocardial Infarction.   Acute myocardial infarction is a self-limited, self-healing disease of the heart that happens also to be a stage in coronary-artery disease. The goal of treatment is to facilitate the healing process, contain the damage to the heart, and protect the patient, if possible, from the sequelae and complications. In many cases the success of therapy is difficult to determine. The success of remedial interventions, such as treatment of heart failure or shock or surgical correction of some major complications, may be judged by the patient's response. But since most therapeutic endeavors are prophylactic, involving attempts to reduce the size of the infarct, prevent ventricular fibrillation, or avert major complications, their effectiveness in individual cases is not known. Evaluation of the success of therapy requires studies comparing results in large samples of treated and untreated patients. Interpretation of data from such intervention trials is often difficult, and the results are occasionally contradictory.

Acute myocardial infarction is in the majority of cases a benign disease. Many patients, even those suffering a large (transmural) myocardial infarction, feel well once the initial attack of chest pain has subsided and make an uneventful recovery. It is even possible to recover without any treatment. For example, occasionally an electrocardiogram taken during a routine checkup of a patient unaware of any heart problem shows unmistakable evidence that he or she has at some time suffered a major myocardial infarction. The initial attack in such a patient may have been milder than usual and have been overlooked or dismissed as an attack of indigestion; consequently the patient continued engaging in normal activity when he or she should have been treated in a hospital.

Nevertheless, the variability of the course of myocardial infarction, together with the possibility of major complications, makes it essential that once the condition is recognized appropriate management be instituted. Treatment is usually initiated in an emergency unit or even during transport of the patient to the hospital. As soon as the probability of myocardial infarction has been established, the patient is moved to the coronary-care unit, first developed in the early 1960s. The expert care in this unit includes electrocardiographic monitoring of the patient's heart rhythm and hemodynamic monitoring in the event of circulatory failure.

Since the risk of serious arrhythmias is highest at the earliest stage of myocardial infarction, monitoring of cardiac rhythm is started as early as possible, in most cases in the ambulance transporting the patient to an emergency unit. Many ambulances are equipped with a transmitter to send electrocardiographic signals to the emergency unit, from where a physician can authorize and direct an ambulance attendant to administer drugs or use defibrillators.

The latest advance in the treatment of myocardial infarction is the use of thrombolytic drugs to dissolve the clot responsible for the infarction. The attack of chest pain usually indicates when a coronary artery became occluded. Death of heart muscle resulting from the occlusion occurs too rapidly to expect that dissolving the clot will prevent myocardial infarction. The basis for thrombolytic therapy rests in the hope that within the first few hours after the occlusion some myocardial cells are still capable of reviving if the blood supply is reestablished, thereby reducing the damage to the heart. Obviously, the earlier the drug is administered, the more likely the patient is to benefit from the treatment. Though this treatment is widely used, a small risk of serious hemorrhage leading to stroke or excessive blood loss calls for caution in administering it to certain patients. An alternative approach to early removal of coronary occlusion is interventional therapy (PTCA) performed immediately after diagnosis. Benefits of thrombolytic treatment have been demonstrated by two major studies, involving observations of thousands of patients, which have shown significant reduction of mortality from myocardial infarction. Benefits from PTCA have not yet been clearly demonstrated; hence its use is still considered experimental. Both approaches are subject to controversy and lively debate among experts regarding which patients are most likely to benefit from such intervention.

Following the initial intervention and after the patient has been moved to the coronary-care unit, management is guided by the patient's condition. Those who feel well and show no significant abnormalities may be transferred within a day or two to a less intensive monitoring facility, then to a regular hospital room, and are candidates for early discharge. Patients who have arrhythmias, unstable blood pressure, or other abnormalities may require longer treatment in each type of facility. Dangerous manifestations, such as heart failure or shock, require intensive therapy, usually guided by hemodynamic monitoring by means of flow-directed cardiac catheters. Cardiogenic shock may require the use of an intraaortic balloon pump.

If chest pain continues beyond the first 24 hours or reappears along with evidence that its origin is ischemic, early coronary angiography may be performed. The results of that test may in turn indicate the need for coronary angioplasty or bypass surgery.

Serious complications of myocardial infarction tend to be delayed; most often they develop between the second and seventh days. Medical staff must be alert to complications at the earliest possible moment since the patient's life may depend on immediate intervention.

Fortunately, most patients will not experience such life-threatening complications and will feel well within 48 hours of the attack. At that point their chance of survival increases to 90–95 percent. The focus of medical management then shifts to rehabilitation. Cardiac rehabilitation in cases of myocardial infarction comprises supervising the patient's gradual resumption of activities and providing psychological support. Myocardial infarction often strikes active, healthy persons without warning, and the prospect of death or disability and uncertainty about the future may have a devastating effect on some patients. Most patients, however, are able to resume a life-style comparable to that prior to the attack, and in many the long-term prognosis is not affected by the attack. Two presidents of the United States, Dwight Eisenhower and Lyndon Johnson, were able to bear the immense stresses of the presidency after recovering from myocardial infarction.

A postinfarction survey of the status of the patient's circulatory system can be performed before discharge from the hospital or, as some physicians prefer, a few weeks later. Prognosis is related to several factors, which can be evaluated by tests: the presence or absence of ischemia as determined by an exercise stress test; the function of the left ventricular pump as determined by echocardiogram or nuclide ventriculogram; and a tendency to precarious ventricular arrhythmias, as determined by a Holter monitor test. The precise battery of tests is tailored to the individual patient. They help the physician decide such questions as whether continuous drug treatment or some intervention (PTCA or bypass surgery) is needed.

Active persons convalescing from myocardial infarction must decide, under guidance from their physician, whether to resume their previous life-style without restrictions, return to their former occupation with some restrictions, retrain for a less strenuous or stressful occupation, or retire. All patients who recover from myocardial infarction should be encouraged to institute or continue preventive measures against atherosclerosis. This secondary prevention involves more aggressive modification of risk factors than does primary prevention. The main emphasis is on reducing cholesterol by diet and, if necessary, drugs. In many patients it is advisable to continue antianginal therapy or other forms of medical therapy.

Sudden Cardiac Death

Coronary-artery disease is the commonest cause of sudden cardiac death (see chap. 7). Sudden death may occur at any stage of coronary disease, but it is a particular concern during and immediately after the initial chest pain of myocardial infarction. In that context it may represent an electrical accident—primary ventricular fibrillation due to instability associated with severe but localized ischemia—or may result from ischemia involving such a large section of the left ventricular muscle as to make survival impossible.

Three patterns of sudden cardiac death (following the one-hour definition) occur in patients with coronary-artery disease:

instantaneous death without warning

cardiac arrest preceded by intermittent or continuous chest pain

cardiac arrest preceded by severe dyspnea including pulmonary edema

Primary ventricular fibrillation is by far the most frequent mechanism of cardiac arrest in these cases. Such patients can usually be resuscitated, and the rate of survival and recovery is good. This response has led some communities to develop programs of widespread training of citizens in cardiopulmonary resuscitation (CPR) for keeping alive someone suffering a heart attack until appropriately equipped medical personnel arrive. Many people have been resuscitated outside the hospital by such means. Studies of survivors of resuscitation reveal that more than half suffered cardiac arrest during the initial stage of myocardial infarction. Among other survivors the arrest was caused by primary ventricular fibrillation resulting from reversible ischemia or was noncoronary in origin. Patients in later stages of coronary-artery disease, particularly those with pump failure, are more difficult to resuscitate and, if successfully resuscitated, have a poor chance of long-term survival.

The most perplexing problem concerns the person with no prior symptoms of coronary-artery disease in whom sudden cardiac death is its first manifestation. Some researchers have attempted to determine whether such apparently healthy persons did indeed have some warning they ignored. Interviews with the families of the deceased revealed that quite a few had sought medical care a short time before the fatal episode. However, symptoms suggesting coronary-artery disease were not always recorded. Since significant symptoms are often ignored, misinterpreted, or subconsciously suppressed, it is possible that warning signs precede sudden cardiac death more often than generally suspected. The available interventions aimed at preventing ventricular fibrillation are limited, yet in a hospital there is a reasonable chance of reviving someone from cardiac arrest— hence the importance of seeking medical care for coronary-artery disease as early as possible.

Chronic Pump Failure

Chronic pump failure, a late stage of coronary-artery disease, results from the destruction of myocardial cells by the recurrent ischemia. In many cases ischemic chest pain is no longer present. Four mechanisms may produce chronic pump failure. (1) A large, transmural myocardial infarction (often leading to left ventricular aneurysm) may affect cardiac function despite survival and recovery from cardiac arrest, so that heart failure persists. (2) Multiple attacks of myocardial infarction can gradually destroy enough heart muscle to cause chronic cardiac failure. (3) Small areas of ischemic damage to the heart muscle, regardless of the presence of myocardial infarction or angina pectoris, may cause heart failure imitating cardiomyopathy (see chap. 10). (4) Mitral insufficiency produced during myocardial infarction may overload the circulation and cause chronic heart failure.

The first two mechanisms account for most cases of chronic pump failure. The actual impairment of cardiac performance does not necessarily determine the amount of disability caused by the heart failure. Despite a low ejection fraction indicative of serious damage, the patient may continue a life free from symptoms, particularly if his or her life-style does not involve strenuous activity. Gradual resumption of activities after myocardial infarction and caution exercised thereafter may prevent the development of dyspnea and other manifestations of heart failure. Nevertheless, significant impairment of cardiac function indicates potential problems even if symptoms are minimal or absent, and the prognosis in such cases is guarded, particularly since patients with impaired left ventricular function are prone to life-threatening ventricular arrhythmias.

Symptomatic patients with chronic pump failure due to coronary-artery disease respond to standard therapy, which may control disability for long periods, especially if the patient is free from angina pectoris. A stable functional impairment of cardiac function without further evidence of ischemia may, with optimal medical management, permit a long life with only a minor effect on its quality. Many other patients, however, suffer from serious disability, developing major complications and even end-stage heart failure, the only remedy for which is cardiac transplantation.

Chapter Nine

Diseases of the Cardiac Valves

The structure of the four cardiac valves is described in chapter 1. To recapitulate their function, the two inflow (atrioventricular) valves—the tricuspid valve on the right side of the heart and the mitral valve on the left—shut to keep blood from backing up into the atria during contraction of the ventricles (systole) and open wide during diastole to permit blood to enter the ventricles from the atria. The two outflow valves—the semilunar valves—separate the ventricles from the large arterial trunks: during diastole the left-sided aortic valve closes off the aorta from the left ventricle, and the right-sided pulmonary valve closes off the right ventricle from the pulmonary artery.

When functioning normally, each valve in the open position permits blood to flow unimpeded through the orifice it protects; to do so, it has to be completely open. In its closed position each valve has to seal the orifice tightly, so as to withstand the pressure difference between the cardiac chambers or great vessels. Thus when a cardiac valve malfunctions, blood may not flow freely through the open orifice or may leak back when the orifice is closed. The former abnormality is called *stenosis* (narrowing) of a valve, the latter *regurgitation* or *insufficiency*.

Both stenosis and regurgitation of cardiac valves have to be considerable to affect the function of the heart. Mild or even moderate stenosis has only a minor effect on the circulation, well within the capability of the heart to adapt. Significant stenosis is usually present when the valve orifice is reduced to less than one-third of its normal size. The narrowed valve then produces resistance to blood flow, which causes pressure to rise in the chamber behind the valve. The consequence of regurgitation is backflow of blood through an incompetent valve; that is, the unidirectional flow of blood becomes bidirectional. Both stenosis and regurgitation increase the workload of the cardiac ventricles.

Rheumatic Fever

An acute disease involving many structures in the body, rheumatic fever particularly afflicts the joints and the heart. Whereas rheumatic disease of the joints heals without aftereffects, involvement of the heart may produce permanent damage to the heart valves; that damage is sometimes immediately apparent, but it may also go undetected for many years. Attacks of rheumatic fever vary in severity; it may manifest itself as an acute, serious disease associated with high fever or appear as minor swelling and pain in the joints. Rheumatic fever is a disease of childhood and in most cases affects persons between the ages of four and twenty.

Though resembling an infectious disease, rheumatic fever is not caused directly by a microorganism. Rather, the body reacts to certain strains of streptococcus (a common bacterium responsible for many different infections, including sore throat) in persons hypersensitive to the microorganism (a process akin to allergy).

The epidemiology of rheumatic fever is one of the more interesting phenomena in contemporary medicine. The prevalence of the disease was high in the United States and other Western countries until the 1950s. Since then its incidence has declined steadily; the cause of this shift is not well understood. By contrast, there has been a dramatic increase in the incidence (or perhaps recognition) of rheumatic fever in third-world countries. As a consequence, rheumatic fever is rarely encountered in the developed countries, whereas in the developing countries of Latin America and Africa and in India it has become the principal cause of heart disease.

A typical attack of rheumatic fever is disabling, producing painful swelling of the large joints—the knees, elbows, and hips—usually migrating from joint to joint and affecting only one at a time. It usually lasts one to four weeks but occasionally persists for months. Involvement of the heart is common but, more often than not, inconspicuous and difficult to detect. Other organs may also be involved, such as the lungs, kidneys, and brain (producing chorea, or uncoordinated movements).

Involvement of the heart appears as *carditis* (also referred to as pancarditis), which consists of rheumatic changes in the three layers of the heart—the endocardium (valves), the myocardium (heart muscle), and the pericardium. Although carditis usually does not affect the function of the heart or produce symptoms, it occasionally brings on serious, even fatal, conditions, such as heart failure, severe incompetence of valves, or large pericardial effusion. Characteristically, changes in the myocardium and pericardium heal without any aftereffects. Rheumatic disease of the valves, however, produces small, wartlike lesions that often initiate a chronic process leading after many years to serious valve disease. The principal damage to heart valves occurs as a result of the healing and scarring of the acute changes. Stenosis of the valve is caused by adhesion between leaflets, incompetence by shrinking of the scarred valve. Thus chronic valve disease is not a direct continuation of the acute disease but usually appears after a long period of apparent complete recovery.

Rheumatic fever has a tendency to recur: a child hypersensitive to streptococcus may suffer an attack each time it is infected. Hence the standard treatment is prophylactic administration of an antibiotic (usually penicillin) to prevent streptococcal infection for many years after the first attack. Recurrence of rheumatic fever increases the severity of valvular disease. In the developing countries, where penicillin prophylaxis is difficult to enforce, children may have yearly attacks of rheumatic fever and develop serious valvular disease at a young age. Thus, though in most cases rheumatic fever is a self-limiting disease, its effect on the cardiac valves may produce disabling heart disease decades later.

Sequelae of Chronic Valvular Disease

Chronic valvular disease involves permanent deformity of a cardiac valve or its neighboring structure. The defect may be congenital (present since birth) or acquired during life in a variety of ways.

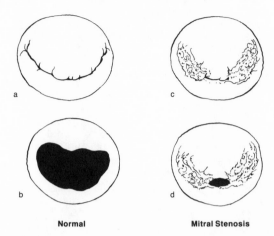

Normal   **Mitral Stenosis**

Figure 31. The mitral valve as seen from the left atrium. (a) Normal mitral valve, closed position, showing two leaflets, one large and one small, covering the orifice completely. (b) Normal mitral valve, open position. (c) Mitral stenosis, closed position, showing the valve with its peripheral portion joined together at the commissures; the central opening still can close completely in systole. (d) Mitral stenosis, open position; during diastole only a small central opening permits blood flow, causing serious obstruction.

Stenosis of a valve, unless congenital, is always the result of a slow process, taking years or decades to reach the point of compromising heart function. Incompetence of a valve can develop abruptly or gradually: it may be caused by a disease of the valve itself, of the ring to which it is attached, or of the auxiliary structures supporting closure of the valve. The two left-sided valves—the mitral and aortic valves—are exposed to pressure several times higher than that exerted on the right-sided valves. The wear and tear on the valves as well as the fact that most cardiac diseases predominantly affect the left ventricle make these two valves more vulnerable. Furthermore, strain on the left ventricle from overload in valvular disease has more serious implications than does strain on the right ventricle.

Stenosis of the mitral valve (fig. 31), when significant, produces resistance to the blood flow during diastole from the left atrium to

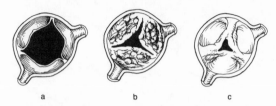

Figure 32. The aortic valve in its open position. (a) Normal valve. (b) Aortic stenosis caused by calcium deposition producing stiffening of the leaflets; the mobility of the valve is limited even though the commissures are free. (c) Aortic stenosis caused by joining together of the peripheral parts of its commissures, similar to mitral stenosis.

the left ventricle. To overcome the resistance and squeeze blood through the narrowed orifice, pressure in the left atrium has to rise (typically to 25 mm Hg instead of the normal 10 mm Hg), whereas the diastolic pressure in the left ventricle, normally identical with that in the atrium, remains unchanged. Mitral stenosis thus produces a pressure gradient across the valve, the magnitude of which depends on the severity of stenosis. High pressure in the left atrium makes the pressure rise in the pulmonary blood vessels, leading to pulmonary hypertension, which in turn overloads the right ventricle and may cause its failure. This mechanical dam at the mitral orifice has an effect on circulation through the lungs similar to that of left ventricular failure (see chap. 5).

Stenosis of the aortic valve (fig. 32) causes resistance of the ejection of blood into the aorta during ventricular systole, which has to be overcome by increased pressure in the left ventricle. Normally during systolic ejection pressures in the left ventricle and the aorta are identical. Aortic stenosis causes a pressure gradient across the aortic valve. For example, in severe aortic stenosis the pressure needed to eject blood into the aorta (which itself has a pressure of 120 mm Hg) may be as high as 240 mm Hg (a gradient of 120 mm Hg), doubling the systolic workload of the left ventricle and leading to its hypertrophy.

In *mitral regurgitation* the left ventricle, while ejecting blood into the aorta, also pumps some blood back into the left atrium. If the volume of backflow is appreciable—sometimes equal to the forward flow into the aorta—the left ventricular workload is significantly increased.

In *aortic regurgitation* the incompetent aortic valve cannot keep blood from being sucked back into the left ventricle during diastole. In severe cases the amount of blood ejected by the left ventricle may be double or triple the normal cardiac output so as to compensate for the backflow, resulting in volume overload and hypertrophy.

In general, then, the effect of valvular disease on the heart is an increase in workload. In contrast to the cardiac consequences of coronary-artery disease, where the heart muscle is damaged and weakened, increased workload produces compensatory hypertrophy of the muscle of the affected ventricle. Thus the cardiac pump becomes stronger than normal, permitting the affected person to lead a normal life for many years. Disability develops late, when hypertrophy of the myocardium can no longer cope with the high workload. Valvular disease is the ideal target for surgical removal of the cause of overload. Not only can surgery correct the disabling symptoms and manifestations of heart failure in such cases, but it may lead to regression of cardiac hypertrophy as well.

The notion of dilating a stenotic mitral valve was expressed as early as 1900, though the means for doing so were not then available. In 1948 surgical technique reached the point where mitral valvotomy could be successfully performed. Throughout the 1950s stenotic valves were dilated by placing fingers or instruments into the beating heart. Mitral stenosis was the most frequent target for so-called closed-heart surgery. Closed mitral valvotomy produced great successes—even today the operation is performed on selected younger patients. (Operations on stenotic aortic and pulmonary valves were less successful and have been abandoned in favor of open-heart repair.)

But during closed operations on a beating heart no actual repair of incompetent valves was possible. The next breakthroughs in valvular surgery came with the introduction of the pump-oxygenator, which made open-heart surgery possible, and then the development of functioning prosthetic valves.

The first successful prosthesis consisted of a plastic ball within a metal cage (fig. 33, left). With the heart stopped, its functions temporarily assumed by the pump-oxygenator, the damaged valve

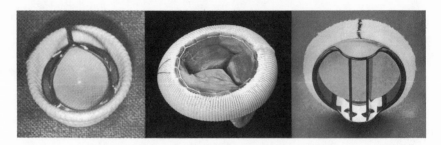

Figure 33. Examples of prosthetic cardiac valves. Left: Prototype mechanical ball valve introduced in the early 1960s. Center: Biological valve taken from a pig's left ventricle mounted on a specially designed ring. Right: A mechanical tilting-disk valve.

was removed and the prosthetic valve sutured into the aortic orifice. Once the heart was restarted, the ball was propelled to the top of the cage by left ventricular contraction, allowing the blood to enter the aorta by passing around it. Ventricular relaxation pulled the ball back into the base, sealing the orifice. A similar ball valve was used to replace faulty mitral valves, with the cage inside the ventricle: ventricular relaxation pulled in the ball and opened the valve, permitting blood to flow from the atrium to the ventricle. Systole forced the ball back to its base, closing the mitral orifice.

Prototype ball valves worked well, with some patients surviving for more than 20 years. Yet the many technical problems and complications spurred the development of new devices. A new approach was introduced a decade after the ball valves, namely the use of biological valves, consisting of human or other animal tissue. The most successful and widely used biological valve is the aortic valve of a pig (porcine heterograft), mounted into a special frame that can be sutured into the mitral or aortic orifice (fig. 33, center). This three-leaflet valve is an ideal substitute for the aortic valve, but it also works well in the mitral position. Modifications of ball valves led to improvements that reduced some of the untoward consequences of the earlier designs. Other prosthetic valves now widely used are fitted with hinged discs to control bloodflow (fig. 33, right).

The major disadvantage of prosthetic valves is that as foreign bodies they are a prime site for the formation of blood clots. These clots may interfere with valvular function, but more often they represent a potential source of emboli, which can cause stroke or other complications. Hence patients with prosthetic valves must remain on anticoagulant therapy throughout their lives. Biological valves greatly reduce the risk of thrombus formation; here anticoagulant treatment is administered only in selected cases. The disadvantage of biological valves, however, is their low durability, for the valve may stiffen and even calcify. The average duration of their normal function is seven to ten years, after which replacement is usually necessary. In children and young adults the process of biological-valve deterioration is greatly accelerated, so that their use in this age group is avoided.

Valvular surgery represents one of the most important advances in the treatment of heart disease, yet there are still many unsolved problems. None of the presently available replacement valves can function as efficiently as the normal natal valve. In addition to clot formation, a number of other complications may develop after successful surgery. And the risk of surgery is not negligible: surgical mortality is estimated at 5–10 percent and may be even greater in high-risk patients. Consequently, deciding the optimal time for valvular surgery is often difficult. Patients in heart failure or seriously disabled by a valvular disease are prime candidates for surgery. Those whose symptoms are still mild enough to allow a reasonably active life may best manage with nonsurgical medical treatment. Early operations in asymptomatic patients aimed at preventing future problems are inadvisable except in special circumstances. In considering candidates for valvular surgery, the physician usually takes into account the patient's occupation and life-style as well as the prognoses with and without surgery.

Clinical Features of Valvular Disease
Mitral Stenosis

Stenosis of the mitral valve is always the aftereffect of acute rheumatic fever. It affects primarily women (60–75 percent of all cases). It takes years for the gradual scarring process following the initial lesions of rheumatic fever to produce mitral stenosis. The interval between the attack (usually in childhood) and the development of symptoms varies widely. One factor is the severity of the attack of rheumatic fever. Furthermore, recurrent attacks lead to more-rapid scarring of the valve. On average, mitral stenosis can first be detected 10 years after the initial attack; significant symptoms may not develop for another 10 to 30 years.

As described in chapter 1, the mitral valve consists of two leaflets separated by two commissures. The initial, rather minor damage to the valve during acute rheumatic fever consists of small lesions located usually at the edges of the leaflet. The healing and scarring process leads to the formation of adhesions between the leaflets, sealing the outer parts of the commissures, so that only the center part of the valve can open during diastole (see fig. 31, p. 129). The normal opening of the mitral orifice during diastole measures 4–6 cm². Only when the sealing process reduces the size of the orifice to less than 2 cm² does the first effect of stenosis develop: the smooth flow of blood through the orifice becomes turbulent, giving rise to a murmur, which the examining physician can detect as evidence of mitral stenosis. However, at this point there is not enough resistance to flow to produce any effect on the circulation. Only further progression of the sealing process leads to the damming up of the orifice, raising the pressure in the left atrium. Usually when the opening is reduced to about 1.5 cm², the patient begins to experience shortness of breath with activity. At this stage (mild mitral stenosis) disability may be minimal, merely requiring the patient to curtail strenuous activities. Sometimes postrheumatic progression stops before symptoms develop, and the patient may go through life without any serious consequences of the disease, in some cases even remaining unaware of its existence. Further progression of mitral stenosis, leaving an orifice of 1 cm² (moderate mitral stenosis), may produce more-pronounced symptoms and disability; furthermore, complications often develop. Severe mitral stenosis (with an orifice of 0.5–0.7 cm²) produces serious disability—congestive heart failure and, in some patients, severe pulmonary hypertension.

Mitral stenosis differs from the other valvular diseases in that the mechanical obstacle to flow occurs *before* the blood enters the left ventricle; hence that important cardiac chamber is spared increased workload. Yet the blood dammed in the left atrium produces an effect on the pulmonary circulation similar to failure of the left ventricle. Consequently, shortness of breath resulting in disability develops early, as soon as mitral stenosis becomes mild or moderate, whereas in the other diseases dyspnea develops late, only when the hypertrophied left ventricle can no longer cope with the overload.

The health of patients with mitral stenosis is frequently affected by complications, which may produce new disabilities or aggravate existing ones:

Atrial fibrillation. Elevated pressure in the left atrium resulting in its dilatation is a powerful contributing factor to atrial fibrillation, present in the majority of patients older than 50 years of age. The onset of atrial fibrillation, as a rule associated with a fast heart rate, is likely to produce disabling dyspnea or heart failure. However, response to treatment is usually satisfactory: as soon as the heart rate is slowed, the patient's symptoms abate or disappear.

Left atrial thrombi with emboli. Atrial fibrillation in the presence of a dilated left atrium facilitates the formation of thrombi attached to the atrial wall. Some portions of the clot may break loose and travel in the bloodstream as emboli, the most serious consequence of which is stroke—a relatively common complication of mitral stenosis. Embolic strokes are often reversible; that is, muscle paralysis and speech disturbance may only be temporary. Some patients, however, may suffer permanently disabling or even fatal strokes in the course of mitral stenosis.

Respiratory infection. Mitral stenosis affects blood flow through the lungs. The resulting congestion facilitates upper respiratory infections. Mild infections are inconsequential, but more-severe infections may greatly increase disability and precipitate heart failure.

Pulmonary hemorrhage. Spitting up of blood occurs commonly in mitral stenosis and is of no significance. Serious hemorrhaging from the lungs, requiring blood transfusion, is rare.

Pulmonary edema. Some patients with mitral stenosis are prone to pulmonary edema, particularly after eating salty food. Though potentially dangerous, pulmonary edema is easily treated, and recurrences can be prevented by restricting dietary salt or administering diuretics.

Severe pulmonary hypertension. In most cases of mitral stenosis elevation of pulmonary arterial pressure is only moderate. But in some patients small pulmonary vessels may react abnormally to elevated pressure in the left atrium by developing severe pulmonary hypertension. This condition seriously compounds disability and may cause intractable heart failure.

Mitral stenosis can generally be diagnosed by performing a physical examination, though evaluation of its severity requires further tests. Among noninvasive tests, electrocardiographic changes and the size and shape of the cardiac shadow in a chest X ray are usually the first indicators in the diagnostic evaluation; an echocardiogram provides further data for estimating the severity of the stenosis and its effect on the circulation. The size of the stenotic mitral orifice can be calculated by means of cardiac catheterization, usually combined with angiography. These two invasive tests are typically performed when surgical treatment is being considered, in which case the extent of pulmonary hypertension and the presence or absence of mitral regurgitation and, in older patients, coronary-artery disease need to be determined.

Surgical repair or replacement of a stenotic mitral valve can not only restore adequate blood flow but also reverse all the secondary effects of mitral stenosis, even in the late stages of the disease. However, several cautionary factors must be considered before deciding on surgery. First, none of the available interventions is capable of restoring fully normal valvular function. Second, early disability in mitral stenosis may be amenable to effective nonsurgical treatment. Third, mitral stenosis often remains stable for years or even permanently, and moderate disability can be controlled by adjustments in life-style. Thus the consensus is that prime candidates for surgery are patients in congestive heart failure or otherwise seriously disabled who are unresponsive to intensive medical treatment.

Several kinds of medical (nonsurgical) treatment are available to patients with mitral stenosis. Diuretics, reinforced by restrictions on salt in the diet, can control fluid retention and the early stages of heart failure. Atrial fibrillation can be treated either by reducing the excessive ventricular rate or by restoring sinus rhythm. To inhibit clot formation, anticoagulants may be administered to certain patients, particularly those experiencing atrial fibrillation. Modification of physical activities may also be recommended.

Surgical treatment of mitral stenosis includes various approaches. In closed mitral valvotomy (without the use of the heart-lung machine) the surgeon introduces a finger (or sometimes a special instrument) into the left atrium of a beating heart to break the adhesions between the two leaflets. This method, the first used in treating mitral stenosis, was the only one available until pump-oxygenators were developed. Open mitral valvotomy (with the use of the heart-lung machine) permits other techniques for separating the leaflets under direct vision. Mitral valvotomy has the advantage of preserving the natal mitral valve and is particularly successful in younger patients in whom the leaflets have not yet stiffened or calcified. A third alternative is replacement of the natal valve with a prosthetic valve or transplanted biological valve. A recent development, invasive but nonsurgical dilatation of the mitral valve (percutaneous balloon mitral valvuloplasty), has been shown to produce satisfactory results in some patients. The long-term effects of this procedure are not yet known.

The dramatic decrease in the incidence of rheumatic fever since the 1940s has greatly reduced the number of cases of mitral stenosis in the Western countries. Most persons in the United States treated for mitral stenosis are over the age of 50; many return for treatment because of the recurrence of stenosis following mitral valvotomy in the distant past or because of malfunction of prosthetic valves. Younger patients with mitral stenosis are mainly immigrants from less-developed countries.

Aortic Stenosis

Stenosis of the aortic orifice is now the commonest valvular disease; it is seen predominantly among the elderly. The term "valvular aortic stenosis" denotes stenosis caused by a stiffened valve and is distinguished from narrowing below or above the aortic valve, occasionally seen as a variety of congenital heart disease.

There are two principal ways in which the aortic valve may become stenotic—fusion of the three valve leaflets, due to adhesion among them, or stiffening and calcification of the leaflets, which may keep the valve from fully opening, leaving a greatly reduced orifice during systole (see fig. 32, p. 130). In addition, aortic stenosis may be present since birth, as a congenital defect in which the three leaflets have grown together, leaving open a small central orifice that can still function normally during diastole.

Acquired fusion of the leaflets by adhesions among them is almost always the result of rheumatic fever and, as in mitral stenosis,
takes decades to develop. Rheumatic aortic stenosis, however, is
now relatively uncommon. Today most cases are considered a type
of "calcific aortic stenosis," a gradual fibrotic thickening of the leaflets in which the deposition of calcium can eventually make the
valve leaflets as hard as bone. Normal leaflets, paper-thin, open
wide in systole, permitting easy flow of blood through the aortic
orifice. The slightest deviation from the norm may alter the flow
patterns through the valve and in time cause minor damage to the
valve. This damage may then produce fibrosis and eventually the
deposition of calcium. A common cause of calcific aortic stenosis is a
minor congenital malformation, namely an aortic valve consisting of
two rather than three leaflets. Such a valve functions normally, and
its presence is seldom recognized. But any minor change in the
shape of the orifice may initiate the process that can produce aortic
stenosis after a period of sixty to seventy years.

Thus aortic stenosis is a disease of old age, with most patients in
their sixties, seventies, or eighties. This process progresses slowly,
so that many years usually elapse from the time aortic stenosis is
first detected until it becomes severe enough to cause symptoms.
The normal aortic orifice during systole measures 3–5 cm^2. When it
reaches about one-half of its normal size, turbulent flow produces a
heart murmur. However, the overload on the left ventricle does not
develop until the orifice is reduced to less than 1.5 cm^2. In moderate
aortic stenosis the orifice has narrowed to 0.7–1.0 cm^2; in severe
aortic stenosis the orifice may be as small as 0.4 cm^2. The degree of
hypertrophy of the left ventricle depends on the severity of stenosis; hence the first manifestation of left ventricular failure may
become apparent only once the stenosis is severe. The patient then
is likely to become aware of shortness of breath during exercise.
Before the onset of left ventricular failure, however, some patients
develop symptoms unique to aortic stenosis, related to the extreme
pressure in the left ventricle and the slow ejection of blood through
the stenotic aortic orifice. Certain reflexes originating in the left
ventricle may interfere with the regulation of blood pressure and
produce sudden loss of consciousness (syncope); furthermore,
blood flow through the coronary arteries may be affected by aortic
stenosis, producing anginalike chest pain unrelated to coronary

disease. Children with congenital aortic stenosis usually tolerate it well, although sometimes unusually severe aortic stenosis may bring about emergencies in infancy.

Aortic stenosis can be detected on physical examination by the characteristic heart murmur and a peculiarity of the pulse. The electrocardiogram will disclose left ventricular hypertrophy, which, though a nonspecific finding, usually indicates that aortic stenosis is at least of moderate severity. In older patients a chest X ray may show calcification of the aortic valve. An echocardiogram can display more directly the narrowing of the aortic orifice, the severity of which can be estimated by the Doppler technique. The size of the aortic orifice can be calculated more accurately from data obtained through cardiac catheterization, which reveals the magnitude of the pressure gradient between the left ventricle and the aorta and the volume of blood flow. In older patients cardiac catheterization is usually combined with coronary angiography. Chest pain, if present, may be caused in these patients by aortic stenosis alone or by coexisting coronary-artery disease—an important distinction when deciding on the proper medical or surgical management of the patient.

In contrast to mitral stenosis, where complications play a major role in its course, there are relatively few complications in aortic stenosis. Atrial and ventricular arrhythmias occasionally develop but are relatively rare. Patients with mitral stenosis are susceptible to infective endocarditis, and preventive measures should be taken. Those with advanced aortic stenosis are at higher risk of sudden cardiac death than those with other valvular diseases.

Treatment of aortic stenosis is almost entirely surgical. Relief of the condition represents one of the most spectacular accomplishments of cardiac surgery and is usually effective even in the most advanced cases. There are several approaches, depending on the type of aortic stenosis. *Aortic commissurotomy*, surgical separation of adherent leaflets through open-heart surgery, is mainly performed on children and adolescents with congenital aortic stenosis. The results are moderately satisfactory, although secondary changes may develop later in life requiring reoperation. *Aortic-valve replacement* is the standard treatment of aortic stenosis. It is the second most frequently performed cardiac operation (after coronary bypass surgery), and its successes are often brilliant: function of the left ventricle, if impaired, returns to normal, and hypertrophy of the left ventricle may regress. *Percutaneous aortic balloon valvuloplasty* has been available only since the mid-1980s; hence its long-range success is uncertain. The advantages of dilating the aortic orifice without surgery are obvious. However, in elderly patients with heavily calcified aortic valves the successful widening of the orifice may not last long, for restenosis is very common. Consequently, this procedure is performed mostly on patients who are poor candidates for open-heart surgery.

The prevailing view is that patients with symptoms clearly related to aortic stenosis should undergo surgery. In the case of an aortic stenosis, even severe, that permits the patient a symptom-free, active life, surgery is usually postponed. Following valve replacement most patients can lead a normal, unrestricted life. Further treatment consists of preventive measures against endocarditis and, in patients with nonbiological valves, anticoagulant therapy. Successful operations are being performed on patients even in their eighties or nineties.

Mitral Regurgitation

The mitral valve is subjected to the highest stresses of the four cardiac valves: it is exposed to the systolic pressure in the left ventricle, at least 120 mm Hg. Its competence is contingent not only on the state and function of its two leaflets but also on the function of the reinforcing auxiliary parts of the mitral-valve apparatus—the chordae tendineae and the papillary muscles of the left ventricle. Consequently, mitral regurgitation may be caused by a variety of mechanisms:

Scarring after rheumatic fever may produce shrinking of the leaflet.

Infective endocarditis may create a hole in a leaflet.

The chordae may stretch, preventing tight closure of the leaflets.

One or more chordae may rupture.

The left ventricular papillary muscle may malfunction and be unable to tighten the chordae.

When the left ventricle dilates, the orifice may become too large for the leaflets to cover it.

The valve may be congenitally deformed.

Mitral regurgitation often develops as a complication of other cardiac diseases. A mild degree of incompetence of this valve has no significant effect on the circulation. Significant mitral regurgitation may also appear as the principal cardiac disease.

Rheumatic mitral regurgitation is most often seen in combination with mitral stenosis, with the latter being the predominant disease. Alone, mitral regurgitation is in some ways similar to mitral stenosis. Although regurgitation in children may be an immediate consequence of rheumatic fever, it is more likely to develop a long time after the attack. Disability tends to appear only in middle age or later. Complications include atrial fibrillation, although embolic episodes are less common than in mitral stenosis. Surgical treatment frequently involves valve replacement, but in some cases the deformed mitral valve can be successfully repaired. In developing countries, where severe recurrent rheumatic fever is prevalent, mitral regurgitation may evolve rapidly, requiring valvular surgery at a young age.

Prolapse of the mitral valve was first identified in the 1960s. Its unique feature is that the volume of blood returning to the left atrium is small and does not increase the workload of the left ventricle. Nevertheless, mitral-valve prolapse has become one of the most widely debated topics in cardiology. The potential complications of this lesion are graver than its direct effect. Mitral-valve prolapse may be associated with the following sequelae:

arrhythmias, both atrial and ventricular

infective endocarditis

embolic stroke (slight but definite risk)

atypical chest pain, which may be mistaken for coronary disease

rupture of some chordae, which can change trivial mitral regurgitation into acute severe mitral regurgitation requiring emergency intervention

In mitral-valve prolapse the leaflets may be larger than normal and stretch the chordae, producing valvular incompetence. Prolapse of the valve means that one leaflet overlaps the other, the most important cause of which is an abnormal structure of the leaflets called mucoid degeneration. This condition is often genetic. Such valves may become progressively larger, with redundant tissues flapping in the mitral orifice like a parachute. Hereditary degeneration of the mitral valve occurs in young patients, is more common in women than in men, and has a relatively high rate of complications. Yet it accounts for only a small fraction of the cases of prolapse. In general, mitral-valve prolapse is a benign condition most frequently discovered on routine examination and having an excellent prognosis.

A preliminary diagnosis of mitral-valve prolapse may be made simply by listening with the stethoscope (auscultation) for the characteristic heart murmur and an extra sound. The principal test used to establish a firm diagnosis of this disease is the echocardiogram, which shows one leaflet slipping over the other. The echocardiogram may in fact be too sensitive a diagnostic tool: normal mitral valves may have somewhat oversized leaflets, which on the echocardiogram may resemble abnormal prolapse. It is now generally recognized that echocardiographic criteria for diagnosing mitral-valve prolapse have to be critically evaluated to guard against ascribing this valvular disease to healthy young adults.

Patients with mitral-valve prolapse need to be reassured of the favorable prognosis. Some patients require endocarditic prophylaxis. Those with the more pronounced hereditary prolapse are sometimes treated for arrhythmias. In rare cases of severe mitral regurgitation valve replacement may become necessary.

Rupture of the chordae tendineae is one of the causes of acute severe mitral regurgitation. It usually develops as a complication of other cardiac diseases, such as mitral-valve prolapse or infective endocarditis, but may represent a primary mitral-valve disease. Spontaneous rupture of the chords occurs occasionally, especially in older male patients. Chordal rupture may also result from trauma, a nonpenetrating injury to the chest. Mild varieties of chordal rupture usually involve separation of a single chord; it may have a minimal hemodynamic effect and require no treatment. More often, however, rupture involves multiple chords and may create an emergency requiring early valve replacement or repair.

Ischemic mitral regurgitation is a complication of coronary-artery disease, most frequently during or after an acute myocardial infarction. It is caused by damage to one of the two papillary muscles in the left ventricle, which then can no longer pull the chordae tendineae tight to help make the valve competent. There are two types. (1) Rupture of the papillary muscle or a part of it is a serious, often catastrophic complication of myocardial infarction and usually requires an emergency valvular operation. (2) Malfunction of a papillary muscle may also develop during the course of myocardial infarction but has less serious consequences. Occasionally mitral regurgitation may not be apparent until after recovery from myocardial infarction. The severity of mitral regurgitation due to damage of the papillary muscle varies; furthermore, regurgitation may become progressively more severe. Treatment may be medical or surgical, depending on the severity of the condition and the patient's response to drug therapy. Valve replacement performed because of heart failure produced by mitral regurgitation may be ineffective if serious postinfarction damage to the heart muscle has occurred.

Infective endocarditis may result in new damage to the mitral valve, causing regurgitation in a previously competent valve. This is sometimes the case in patients with mitral stenosis or when the infection develops on a valve with a minor abnormality not affecting its function, such as mitral-valve prolapse. If the infection is seated on an already incompetent valve, the amount of regurgitation may increase, particularly if infection produces perforation of the valve or disrupts the chordae tendineae. Acute mitral regurgitation caused by endocarditis, if severe, may lead to a cardiac emergency requiring immediate valvular surgery.

Rarer varieties of mitral regurgitation include congenital mitral valve clefts (division of one or both leaflets into two parts with a space between them), marked dilatation of the left ventricle in association with heart failure, and cardiac tumors (myxomas of the left atrium), which may interfere with the closure of the valve.

Aortic Regurgitation

There are several causes of incompetence of the aortic valve:

rheumatic damage to the leaflets

perforation of leaflets in infective endocarditis

disease of the aortic root (the initial portion of the aorta just above the valve)

congenital deformity (either combined with other malformations or
  as a sole lesion)

trauma producing detachment of a leaflet

Two basic mechanisms produce aortic regurgitation—abnormality
of the leaflet and dilatation of the root of the aorta (the ring to which
the valve is attached becomes widened and the orifice too large for
healthy valves to cover it).

Given a comparable volume of blood regurgitating through an
incompetent left-sided cardiac valve, aortic regurgitation imposes a
greater overload on the left ventricle than does mitral regurgitation. Blood leaking through an incompetent mitral valve into the
atrium raises the left ventricular workload mildly; blood returning
to the left ventricle through an incompetent aortic valve has to be
ejected again into the aorta, steeply increasing the workload. This
difference results in a more pronounced hypertrophy of the left
ventricle in aortic regurgitation. Furthermore, the large volume of
blood handled by the left ventricle dilates it. The dilated, volume-
overloaded left ventricle characteristic of aortic regurgitation works
less efficiently than the nondilated, pressure-overloaded left ventricle in aortic stenosis.

In the past, chronic aortic regurgitation was caused frequently
by rheumatic fever, with or without coexisting mitral stenosis.
With the decline in the prevalence of rheumatic heart disease in
the West, the commonest cause of chronic aortic regurgitation has
become disease of the aortic root, a variety of aortitis affecting the
portion of the aorta immediately above the aortic valve (see chap.
14). Syphilitic aortitis was once common, often affecting the aortic
valve, but today it is a rarity. Nowadays aortitis may be associated
with certain varieties of rheumatoid arthritis or may develop as a
result of atherosclerotic disease of the aorta in the elderly.

On physical examination aortic regurgitation displays a characteristic heart murmur. The severity of the regurgitation can be estimated by abnormalities of the arterial pulse and unusually low
diastolic blood pressure. Aortic insufficiency cannot be quantified,
but a more accurate estimation of regurgitant volume is possible by
echocardiography, using the Doppler principle. As a rule, cardiac
catheterization contributes little to the diagnosis.

The consequences of aortic regurgitation depend on whether the lesion develops gradually or abruptly. The increased workload acute aortic regurgitation imposes on a normal left ventricle, if severe, may produce life-threatening heart failure requiring emergency valvular surgery. Chronic aortic regurgitation, by contrast, permits adaptive hypertrophy of the ventricle and is generally well tolerated; patients with severe aortic regurgitation may lead an unrestricted active life for many years. Eventually the left ventricle reaches the limit of its adaptative capacity, leading to cardiac failure. But in aortic regurgitation, more than in other valvular diseases, the onset of the first symptoms (usually dyspnea produced by activity) may develop so late that relief of the overload by valve replacement may no longer restore good left ventricular function. To avert this problem, in aortic regurgitation early deterioration of left ventricular function is occasionally considered an indication for surgery even in asymptomatic patients. When symptoms suggestive of heart failure are present, surgery is mandatory.

The major complication of aortic regurgitation is infective endocarditis. Atrial fibrillation is rare; ventricular arrhythmias may appear during late stages. The prolonged asymptomatic course of aortic regurgitation usually makes medical treatment unnecessary except to prevent endocarditis.

Other Diseases of the Cardiac Valves

Pulmonary stenosis is almost always congenital. It will be discussed in chapter 10. *Pulmonary regurgitation* is rare. It occasionally develops in severe pulmonary hypertension, without intrinsic disease of the valve leaflets, when high pressure in the pulmonary artery makes the healthy pulmonary valve incompetent. Damage to the pulmonary valve may occur in infective endocarditis, found most frequently in intravenous drug abusers since bacteria introduced with intravenously administered drugs tend to infect right-sided cardiac valves.

Tricuspid stenosis is a rare complication of rheumatic fever. It almost always coexists with mitral-valve disease. *Tricuspid regurgitation* is a relatively common sequel to pulmonary hypertension. It commonly results in right ventricular failure, when the tricuspid orifice stretches, making the valve incompetent. Its presence merely aggravates the effect of right ventricular failure on the pressure in the veins bringing blood to the right atrium. Tricuspid-valve repair or replacement is occasionally imperative, but physicians prefer to avoid it because operations on the tricuspid valve are not as effective as those performed on left-sided cardiac valves. Tricuspid-valve involvement may also occur in endocarditis among drug abusers.

Combined diseases of cardiac valves are a relatively common consequence of rheumatic fever involving the mitral and aortic valves. Aortic stenosis or regurgitation resulting from rheumatic fever is more frequent in combination with mitral-valve involvement (usually stenosis) than as the sole consequence of rheumatic fever. The course and prognosis of double valve disease usually follows the pattern of the predominant lesion.

Stenosis of the mitral or aortic valve may be associated with incompetence of the same valve. The consequences of combined stenosis and regurgitation of a left-sided cardiac valve usually differ little from those of pure stenosis; less commonly, however, they follow the pattern of pure regurgitation of the valve.

Infective Endocarditis

The term "infective endocarditis" has replaced the older term "subacute bacterial endocarditis." It is the most serious complication of valvular heart disease, an infection of the cardiac valves caused most often by bacteria and occasionally by fungi but not by viruses. Cardiac valves are not the only sites of infection; congenital heart lesions are also susceptible. It is unusual for endocarditis to develop on healthy valves since microorganisms tend to settle on damaged endocardium.

Bacteria in the bloodstream (bacteremia) is common even in health. A variety of organisms normally present on the skin and in the mouth, nose, and rectum may enter the bloodstream as a result of minor cuts or punctures. The body's defense mechanisms take care of eliminating the bacteria unless they can find a vulnerable spot in the inner lining of the heart and blood vessels; even then only occasionally can they take sufficient hold to cause infection. Certain conditions or procedures are likely to introduce large numbers of microorganisms into the bloodstream and thus carry a higher-than-average risk of starting an infection:

dental surgery

surgical procedures or manipulations involving the gastrointestinal and genitourinary tracts

intravenous injection of drugs among drug abusers

superficial infections such as abscesses

Invasion of microorganisms into a damaged endocardium produces a local reaction. Blood cells accumulate, including platelets and fibrin, which along with small thrombi form a structure, called a vegetation, that attaches itself to the valve. Single vegetations have the appearance of small pearls, but they tend to aggregate, producing larger structures sometimes resembling a bunch of small grapes. These vegetations can damage valvular tissue by producing holes in the valves or actually chewing up portions of them. Moreover, they may detach themselves and float away in the bloodstream, producing emboli. The consequences of infection of valves and the extent of damage are related to the type of microorganism, its aggressiveness (virulence), the extent of blood contamination, and the time antibiotic therapy is started.

The onset of endocarditis may be sudden, characterized by chills and high fever (acute endocarditis). More often, however, endocarditis develops inconspicuously and may not be recognized for weeks or even months (subacute endocarditis). In such cases patients may be aware of a certain lassitude or lack of pep. Fever is almost always present, though it may be slight. Anemia often accompanies subacute endocarditis. The correct diagnosis is frequently apparent, despite the vague symptoms, if the patient is known to be at risk for endocarditis because of valvular or congenital heart disease. However, if the presence of heart disease is undetected—as in the case of trivial valvular lesions—considerable difficulties may arise in interpreting the symptoms.

Endocarditis affects patients in several ways. The infection may spread and cause death. (The mortality rate from endocarditis is about 20 percent.) The destructive process on valves may produce acute, severe valvular regurgitation, leading to heart failure or even shock. Loose vegetations may produce embolic damage to distant organs such as the brain, kidneys, or spleen. Prompt antibiotic therapy can cure the infection without any aftereffects.

Infective endocarditis is suspected in cases of unexplained fever in patients with valvular or congenital heart lesions. A more direct clue to the diagnosis is a heart murmur not present previously. Also of aid in diagnosing the disease is echocardiography, which can detect vegetations provided they have reached significant size. The confirmatory test is a blood culture to identify the organism responsible for the infection. A sample of the patient's blood is placed in a medium, such as broth, on which bacteria thrive and is incubated at body temperature. Once the organism has been identified, the proper antibiotic therapy can be chosen and the prognosis determined.

The commonest cause of subacute infective endocarditis is the green streptococcus (*Streptococcus viridans*). But almost every known microorganism capable of invading the body can, under appropriate circumstances, produce endocarditis. Some of them can be cultured and identified within 24 to 48 hours. Others may need special culture mediums and techniques. In 10–20 percent of cases the infecting organism cannot be identified.

Antibiotic therapy is required for all cases of infective endocarditis and is started as soon as the microorganism is identified. If prompt identification from blood culture is not forthcoming, interim therapy with some broadly effective antibiotics should be administered. The effect of therapy is often apparent within a few days, as the fever and malaise disappear; however, antibiotic therapy should be continued for a few weeks after the symptoms have passed, to ensure that all viable infecting organisms have been eliminated from the body. The initial therapy is usually administered intravenously and is later replaced by oral antibiotics. Follow-up blood cultures help in monitoring the success of treatment.

Whether therapy other than antibiotics is indicated depends on the extent of damage to the valves or other infected structures. Endocarditis caused by the green streptococcus is relatively benign and usually requires only antibiotic therapy. Fungi, yeasts, and more-aggressive bacteria may cause extensive valvular damage, often requiring surgical removal of the infected valve and its replacement with a prosthesis. In an emergency such as severe heart failure the surgery may be performed despite the infection, but it is preferable to wait until the organisms are destroyed by antibiotics.

Prosthetic valves themselves can be targets of bacterial infection; infected prostheses usually require replacement.

Preventive therapy should be undertaken in all patients at risk of infective endocarditis. It consists of administering an antibiotic before procedures that may introduce microorganisms into the bloodstream and continuing treatment briefly thereafter. Among conditions requiring antibiotic prophylaxis are dental extractions and surgery, diagnostic and therapeutic procedures in the gastrointestinal and genitourinary tracts, and childbirth. Antibiotic prophylaxis does not offer total protection but does reduce the probability of infecting the heart.

Chapter Ten

Diseases of the
Myocardium and Pericardium

Diseases of the Myocardium

This chapter deals with rarer varieties of heart muscle disease caused by conditions other than coronary disease. The life-sustaining function of the heart depends on the pumping capacity of the left ventricular heart muscle, and, to a lesser extent, that of the right ventricular muscle. The commonest cause of impairment of left ventricular function is destruction of heart muscle cells produced by myocardial ischemia as a part of coronary disease (see "Pump Failure," chapter 8).

Acute Myocarditis

Any inflammatory process affecting the heart muscle is referred to as *myocarditis*. In most cases myocarditis results from an infection, although there are other causes as well. Involvement of the myocardium occurs commonly in some acute infectious diseases, especially those caused by viruses; but owing to the benign nature of myocarditis, it routinely goes unrecognized.

Many viral childhood diseases—mumps, measles, poliomyelitis—may lead to myocarditis. As a rule, they do not produce any symptoms, and hence the myocarditis cannot be recognized on physical examination; its presence can only be detected by special tests. Since it usually has no significant sequelae, testing for myocarditis is not indicated. However, in rare cases myocarditis may lead to heart failure and even death. It is believed that myocarditis is principally responsible for the rare deaths from influenza. In the past, when diphtheria was common, myocarditis due to a toxin of the diphtheria bacillus was a dreaded complication of that disease. Myocarditis may coexist with viral pericarditis, to be discussed later in this chapter. It can also be caused by some drugs and by radiation therapy. As a part of the hypersensitivity mechanism, myocarditis is often a manifestation of diseases related to allergic reaction, such as acute rheumatic fever. Myocardial involvement occurs occasionally in infectious mononucleosis, viral hepatitis, and Lyme disease.

Even in those rare cases where heart failure results from acute myocarditis, complete recovery is the commonest outcome. Occasionally viral myocarditis may initiate dilated cardiomyopathy (see below). Heart failure caused by myocarditis may persist beyond the acute stage, turning into dilated cardiomyopathy. More often, however, there is an apparent recovery from acute myocarditis, with cardiomyopathy developing gradually months or years later. The possibility that some cases of dilated cardiomyopathy of unknown cause may also be the consequence of past, unrecognized myocarditis has been suggested, though not proved.

Clinically significant acute myocarditis presents itself usually by the onset of dyspnea. Signs of heart failure appear without obvious cause but are often associated with a fever. Diagnostic studies may show electrocardiographic abnormalities, which are particularly significant if day-to-day changes are observed. Chest X ray may reveal enlargement of the heart shadow. Echocardiography and nuclide ventriculogram are the definitive tests for determining the degree to which ventricular function is impaired.

Because of the self-limiting nature of myocarditis, in most cases no treatment is necessary. If a contributive allergic factor is suspected, the use of immunosuppressive drugs, including corticosteroids, may be justified.

The Cardiomyopathies

Cardiomyopathy refers to a variety of conditions involving chronic disease of the heart muscle. There are three categories of cardiomyopathy:

dilated (congestive) cardiomyopathy

hypertrophic cardiomyopathy

restrictive cardiomyopathy

Dilated cardiomyopathy is the commonest type. It is characterized by dilation of the left ventricle associated with its impaired
performance, which can range from minor functional disturbance
to intractable heart failure. Dilated cardiomyopathy is the result of
various factors damaging the heart muscle. As a primary disease of
the myocardium unrelated to cardiac overload, dilated cardiomyopathy is not associated with hypertrophy of cardiac ventricles.

Most cases of dilated cardiomyopathy develop as a primary disease without an identifiable cause (idiopathic cardiomyopathy). As
mentioned, some cases may represent late aftereffects of viral
myocarditis. The onset of cardiomyopathy is usually inconspicuous
(unless it is a continuation of acute myocarditis). The first symptoms
are typically mild and nondisabling. Progression to disability may
take many years, though occasionally the process moves rapidly.

In some cases dilated cardiomyopathy may have an identifiable
cause or be associated with special situations. Myocardial damage
may result from heavy alcohol abuse (alcoholic cardiomyopathy).
Drugs or chemical substances may do permanent damage to the
heart muscle (toxic cardiomyopathy). For example, in 1960 in the
Great Lakes region of the United States and Canada an epidemic of
cardiomyopathy was traced to cobalt mixed into the beer to stabilize the foam. Certain drugs used in chemotherapy to treat cancer
exert a toxic effect on the heart. Cardiomyopathy related to childbirth (peripartum cardiomyopathy) is a rare complication that may
develop during the last trimester of pregnancy or after delivery.
Cardiomyopathy may also develop in the course of coronary-artery
disease (see chap. 8).

The first symptom of dilated cardiomyopathy patients become
aware of is shortness of breath. Tolerance for exercise may gradually
decrease until other evidence of heart failure develops. Yet cardiomyopathy may be discovered by a physician before any symptoms
are present. Changes in the electrocardiogram taken during a routine checkup, discovery of an arrhythmia, or cardiac enlargement on
X-ray examination may trigger further cardiac evaluation. A finding
of reduced contraction of either or both ventricles, demonstrated by

echocardiography or nuclide ventriculography, is central to the diagnosis (so long as there is no evidence of coronary-artery disease or valvular malfunction). Biopsy of the heart muscle by means of cardiac catheterization may be performed if unusual varieties of cardiomyopathy amenable to drug therapy are suspected.

No specific therapy for cardiomyopathy is available, except in rare cases where response to corticosteroids may be anticipated. The results of conventional treatment of heart failure vary. In many cases a disability can be managed for years. Yet deterioration into end-stage heart failure is inevitable. The only type of cardiomyopathy in which a complete regression of the disease is possible is peripartum cardiomyopathy.

Complications of cardiomyopathy include ventricular arrhythmias and intracardiac thrombi, possible sources of emboli. Treatment of complications includes the use of anticoagulants to prevent intracardiac thrombi and antiarrhythmic drugs to control serious ventricular arrhythmias. Dilated cardiomyopathy is the commonest indication for cardiac transplantation.

Hypertrophic cardiomyopathy is a hypertrophy, or excessive development, of the myocardium of the left ventricle, or both ventricles, without a corresponding increase in cardiac workload. Examination of the heart muscle in this condition under the microscope reveals abnormal structure of muscle fibers, which appear disorganized and thicker and larger than normal. The cause of hypertrophic cardiomyopathy is not known, but it often runs in families and in those cases may be due to a genetic error. Hypertrophic cardiomyopathy affects people of all ages; the hereditary variety may manifest itself in adolescents and young adults.

In contrast to work hypertrophy found in valvular and other cardiac diseases, hypertrophy in this variety of cardiomyopathy is not evenly distributed throughout the muscle of the left ventricle but affects primarily the cardiac septum, which bulges into the cavity of the left ventricle or, less commonly, both ventricles. This selective thickening of the septum is most frequent at its upper part, close to the mitral valve, and may obstruct the flow of blood ejected during systole into the aorta. The abnormal bulge can also interfere with the mitral leaflets, creating resistance to outflow from the left ventricle, much as in aortic stenosis, which results in abnormally high pressure in the left ventricle. As a further consequence, the mitral valve, now in an abnormal position, may become incompetent. These abnormalities of outflow from the left ventricle produce symptoms in some patients, namely chest pain similar to angina pectoris and attacks of sudden weakness, dizziness, or syncope.

Manifestations of hypertrophic cardiomyopathy vary greatly. Many patients remain asymptomatic for years and often survive to old age. Symptoms, if present, may appear episodically or with disabling frequency. They can usually be controlled by drugs; if drugs prove ineffective, surgical treatment is also available. However, the condition does carry a risk of sudden cardiac death, assumed to be due to fatal arrhythmias.

Complications of hypertrophic cardiomyopathy include atrial and ventricular arrhythmias. There is some risk of stroke from systemic emboli, almost always associated with complicating atrial fibrillation. Mitral regurgitation, frequently present, is usually inconsequential, although in rare cases severe mitral regurgitation may necessitate mitral-valve replacement. There is also a small risk of infective endocarditis.

The diagnosis of hypertrophic cardiomyopathy, often suggested by physical examination, is definitively established by echocardiography, which displays the thickened septum and the abnormal motion of the mitral valve. Treatment of hypertrophic cardiomyopathy includes the use of drugs to reduce the force of left ventricular contraction, thereby reducing the obstruction. These include beta-adrenergic blocking agents and calcium channel blockers. Surgery is reserved for severely symptomatic patients unresponsive to medical therapy. It consists of resecting a portion of the hypertrophic septum located opposite the mitral valve to eliminate or greatly reduce the outflow obstruction and relieve symptoms. There are, however, disadvantages to surgical therapy: first, the desired effects are not always attainable; second, the average mortality of the procedure is higher than for valvular surgery; third, there is no definite evidence that successful operations influence longevity.

Restrictive cardiomyopathy is the rarest of the three cardiomyopathies. Unlike dilated cardiomyopathy, in restrictive cardiomyopathy the left ventricle is of normal size and contracts normally; however, the disease affects its relaxation. Thus inadequate cardiac output is related to deficient filling; that is, not enough blood enters the ventricle. Dilated cardiomyopathy is caused by systolic ventricular malfunction, restrictive cardiomyopathy by diastolic ventricular malfunction. In other words, dilated hearts cannot empty, and stiff hearts cannot fill. At rest the affected ventricle accepts the normal amount of blood; but during periods of increased activity the needed additional blood remains in the left atrium. Hence pressure in that chamber may rise in diastole, producing a chain of sequelae in the pulmonary circulation identical to that of congestive cardiac failure.

Restrictive cardiomyopathy is most frequently caused by diseases infiltrating the heart and other organs, such as amyloidosis, sarcoidosis, and hemosiderosis. Inadequate diastolic filling of the ventricles occurs also in constrictive pericarditis (see below), and it is often difficult to determine which of the two conditions is the cause of diastolic heart failure in a given case.

Patients with restrictive cardiomyopathy develop shortness of breath, which may progress to congestive heart failure. Diagnosis follows a finding of congestive heart failure despite a normal ventricular ejection fraction and normal-sized heart. Definitive identification of its cause can often be made on the basis of a myocardial biopsy.

Diseases of the Pericardium

As explained in chapter 1, the pericardium consists of two layers of a thin membrane, one lining the outside of the heart (visceral pericardium), the other enveloping the heart and the first portions of the great vessels (parietal pericardium). Between the two layers is space for a small amount of fluid acting as a lubricant to reduce friction between them during cardiac motion. An increase in the amount of pericardial fluid (pericardial effusion) occurs in many conditions affecting the heart and other organs. The parietal pericardium has enough elasticity to accommodate a fair amount of pericardial fluid, so that pericardial effusion ordinarily does not interfere with the function of the heart.

Diseases of the pericardium may have a significant effect on the function of the heart if they restrict its motion. Restriction can develop if the amount of pericardial fluid exceeds the elastic capacity of the parietal pericardium or if the pericardium thickens and loses its elasticity.

Pericardial tamponade occurs if pericardial fluid accumulates too rapidly to permit adaptive stretching of the pericardium. The pressure in the pericardial sac rises, and when it exceeds that in the atria, the filling of the heart in diastole is interfered with. Tamponade is a serious condition that may become a life-threatening emergency. Though tamponade may develop in the course of acute pericarditis, its most dangerous cause is the escape of blood from the heart into the pericardial sac, a condition known as hemopericardium. The principal cause of naturally occurring hemopericardium is rupture of the heart during acute myocardial infarction. This complication is usually fatal, although occasionally there is enough time to perform immediate corrective surgery. The commonest cause of pericardial tamponade due to hemopericardium is trauma resulting from one of the many diagnostic or therapeutic intracardiac interventions and, rarely, from cardiac surgery. Tamponade may also develop because of external trauma—stab wounds or gunshot wounds.

The immediate consequence of tamponade is a fall in arterial blood pressure and an increase in venous pressure. When arterial pressure reaches shock level, tamponade becomes a life-threatening emergency and must be recognized immediately. Instant relief follows removal of blood or fluid from the pericardium by means of a needle inserted through the skin and the chest wall into the pericardial sac. It is sometimes necessary to supplement this treatment with surgical drainage of the pericardium.

Acute pericarditis is most often caused by viral infection either as a part of general infection with a virus or as a disease limited to the pericardium. It is usually a self-limiting febrile illness lasting one to two weeks and almost never has immediate aftereffects. The principal feature of acute pericarditis is chest pain, which may resemble the ischemic pain of coronary-artery disease. In rare cases fluid accumulation may be rapid enough to produce tamponade. The diagnosis of pericarditis is commonly made on the basis of characteristic abnormalities in the electrocardiogram. However, the most sensitive and reliable means of demonstrating pericardial fluid is echocardiography.

Acute pericarditis is treated with antiinflammatory drugs to control the pain. Although acute pericarditis is often referred to as benign, in a small number of cases there are late consequences. One or more attacks of recurrent pericarditis may develop at intervals of a few weeks. Late appearance of constrictive pericarditis (see below) may take place particularly in patients who have had more than one attack.

Acute pericarditis similar to the viral variety often develops from one of the systemic diseases characterized by an allergic-type reaction. These diseases include rheumatic fever, systemic lupus erythematosus, and rheumatoid arthritis. Pericarditis can also occur after acute myocardial infarction (Dressler syndrome) and occasionally after cardiac surgery (postcardiotomy syndrome). These attacks are particularly prone to recur periodically.

Chronic pericardial effusion may develop with or without disease of the pericardium. Increased fluid in the pericardial sac is common in cases of general fluid retention due to cardiac or renal disease. As such it produces no symptoms and may be discovered by chest X ray (marked enlargement of the cardiac shadow) or echocardiography. When pericardial disease is present, persistence of fluid is often a precursor of constrictive pericarditis. *Tuberculous pericarditis* is characterized by pericardial effusion persisting for years and gradually leading to thickening of the pericardium and pericardial constriction, with eventual disappearance of the fluid. *Uremic pericarditis* is a common complication of chronic kidney failure; tamponade and, rarely, constrictive pericarditis may result. *Neoplastic pericarditis* may be caused by primary tumors (neoplasms) of the pericardium or by invasion of tumors from elsewhere, particularly the lungs. *Postradiation pericarditis* may develop in patients after radiotherapy for cancer in the chest, including breast cancer.

Echocardiography is the principal diagnostic tool in pericardial effusion. Frequently a pericardial needle tap (to remove fluid) is needed to determine the nature of the effusion, particularly if tuberculosis or neoplasm is suspected. Surgical drainage or removal of parts of the pericardium may be indicated even in the absence of fully developed constrictive pericarditis.

Chronic constrictive pericarditis is present when a diseased pericardium becomes so thick and stiff that the filling of the heart is interfered with. The two layers of the pericardium often adhere to each other, forming a firm, inelastic structure in which the heart is encased. In late stages of constrictive pericarditis calcium deposits may envelop the heart in a bonelike armor. Constrictive pericarditis often resembles congestive heart failure. But because of its chronicity massive edema and enlargement of the liver, which may result in secondary cirrhosis of the liver, are much more common than in congestive heart failure.

At one time, most cases of constrictive pericarditis were caused by tuberculosis, which today is rare. Now constriction may be the end result of acute pericarditis and may sometimes be found in cases of uremic pericarditis and neoplastic pericarditis. It is also a complication of radiation therapy for cancer of the breast or other structures in the chest. The diagnosis of constrictive pericarditis can often be made on the basis of physical examination and X rays. Echocardiography is helpful but may not be as decisive as in pericardial effusion. As mentioned, it is occasionally difficult to distinguish constrictive pericarditis from restrictive cardiomyopathy. Treatment is primarily surgical, although in early stages diuretics can provide considerable relief of symptoms. Surgical removal of the thick pericardium does not require that the heart be opened; nevertheless, the risk in surgery is moderately high.

Purulent pericarditis involves the accumulation of pus in the pericardial space. It frequently is a complication of a purulent process in the chest. This type of pericarditis usually requires prolonged surgical drainage.

Chapter Eleven

Congenital Heart Disease

Many imperfections may be found in the heart of a newborn. In approximately 1 percent of live births there is a significant malformation of the heart that may affect the child's health. Such congenital defects may be restricted to the heart or may also show up in other organs and parts of the body. These malformations fall into three groups:

defects having no effect on the function of the heart or on the development of the child but sometimes leading to problems later in life (such as a bicuspid aortic valve)

defects affecting the function of the heart but compatible with normal or near-normal development and survival to adulthood

defects incompatible with survival beyond infancy

In some cases the cause of the defect can be identified. Genetic and environmental factors may be responsible for malformations of a fetus. Genetic errors involving identifiable chromosomal abnormalities usually produce multiorgan syndromes (the best known is Down's syndrome), which frequently involve the heart; genetic errors affecting the heart alone sometimes appear in several members of a family. However, genetic factors account for only about 8 percent of cases of congenital malformation of the heart. Certain environmental agents cause congenital cardiac malformations if the mother is exposed to them during the early stages of pregnancy. These include viral infections (particularly maternal German measles), drugs, tobacco, and alcohol. Malnutrition of the mother can also lead to such defects.

The effect of cardiac birth defects on the function of the heart and circulation is related to two basic factors—stenosis of various points of the circulation (usually cardiac orifices or the aorta) and abnormal communication between the two sides of the circulation. Abnormal openings or ducts connecting the arterial and venous sides of the circulation are unique to congenital heart disease, and their size and location usually determine the seriousness of the malformation.

The normal pathway of fetal circulation is illustrated in figure 34. The principal difference between the fetal circulation and the circulation after birth is that in the former the process of acquiring oxygen and disposing of carbon dioxide takes place in the mother's placenta rather than in the lungs. During the second and third trimesters of pregnancy all the tissues of the body are formed and require a steady supply of oxygen. Oxygenated blood from the mother's placenta enters the fetal inferior vena cava through the umbilical vein and hence into the right side of the heart. From there part of the blood enters the left atrium through the *foramen ovale*, and the rest is propelled into the pulmonary artery. But instead of flowing into the inactive lungs, most of this remainder is directed into the descending aorta through a special duct, the *ductus arteriosus*. Whereas in the permanent postnatal circulation fully oxygenated "pink" blood fills the systemic arterial system and the deoxygenated "blue" blood the systemic venous system (each totally separate), the fetus lives on a mixture of oxygenated and deoxygenated blood. Oxygenated blood from the placenta and deoxygenated blood returning from the fetus's body are mixed in the right atrium and shunted into the left side of the heart, supplying the head and upper extremities. Most of the blood ejected into the pulmonary artery is deflected through the ductus arteriosus into the descending aorta, supplying the lower part of the body. The tissues of the fetus adapt to the lower oxygen content of this blood, although it gives the outward appearance of the fetus a purplish tinge.

After birth the two fetal structures permitting communication between the two sides of the circulation—the foramen ovale and the ductus arteriosus—close, but in some cases they may remain

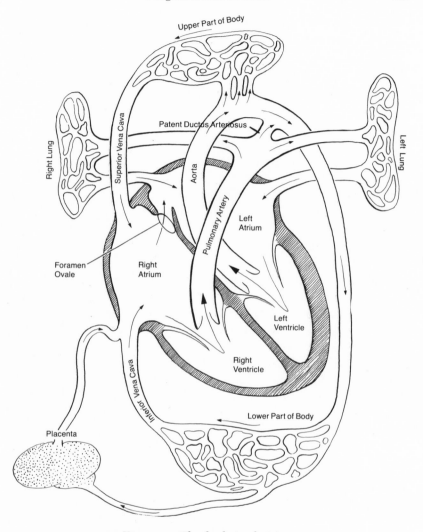

Figure 34. The fetal circulation.

open, providing an abnormal pathway for blood mixing. In addition, other abnormal communications may permit blood mixing as a result of fetal malformation.

The mixing of fully oxygenated arterial blood and deoxygenated venous blood is a unique feature of some congenital cardiac malformations. When the admixture of venous blood in the arteries reaches a certain level it results in *cyanosis*, a purplish or bluish discoloration of the skin and lips. Temporary cyanosis, particularly of the extremities, is a common phenomenon in healthy subjects, for whenever the circulation through a part of the body slows down (for example, because of exposure to cold or the placement of a tourniquet), more oxygen is extracted from the blood by the tissues. Slowed circulation in patients who are in heart failure may produce cyanosis of the entire body. Under these conditions the arterial blood is fully oxygenated, but the oxygen content of the venous blood is unusually low (*peripheral cyanosis*). In *central cyanosis*, however, it is the arterial blood that contains a reduced amount of oxygen; its most common cause is blood mixing. Another mechanism of central cyanosis is deficient oxygen exchange in the lungs in some pulmonary diseases.

Blood mixing in congenital heart disease occurs in one of two ways: as a shunt, when a certain volume of deoxygenated blood enters the left side of the heart or the aorta, or as complete mixing (analogous to fetal circulation), when the arterial and venous blood mix freely in some part of the heart. Either mechanism results in reduced oxygen saturation of the arterial blood. Normal oxygen saturation is at least 95 percent; small or moderate shunts may reduce oxygen saturation to 85–90 percent. The normal extraction of oxygen by tissues remains unchanged when arterial oxygen saturation is reduced; hence oxygen saturation of the venous blood drops. Large shunts or free mixing of blood may reduce arterial oxygen saturation to as low as 60 percent. Cyanosis in infants, colloquially termed "blue baby," becomes visible at an oxygen saturation level of about 85 percent, though the threshold can vary widely.

Cardiovascular shunts allow the flow of blood through an abnormal opening or duct between the arterial and venous circulations. Intracardiac shunts result from defects in the atrial or ventricular septum; a common extracardiac shunt is due to a persistent fetal ductus arteriosus. In the postnatal circulation the pressure in the left heart chambers or the aorta is higher than in the corresponding parts of the right heart and pulmonary artery; hence the usual direction of the shunts is into the right side of the circulation (*left-to-right shunt*). When the fully oxygenated blood in the left heart and aorta reenters the right side, there is no effect on oyxgen saturation of either arterial or venous blood. Under abnormal circumstances shunting may occur in the opposite direction (*right-to-left shunt*), in which case lower oxygen saturation and cyanosis develop.

Narrowing of the cardiac orifices may involve the valves (*congenital valvular stenosis*) or other structures where blood flows into and out of the heart. A relatively common malformation is stenosis of the aorta at a point where the aortic arch joins the descending aorta (*coarctation of the aorta*).

The complexity of congenital malformations of the heart, particularly in infants, presents a challenge in establishing the correct diagnosis. Some of the simpler defects can be recognized in infancy by the presence of heart murmurs. Intracardiac communications may cause the blood flow through the abnormal defect to be turbulent, thereby producing a murmur. Murmurs of ventricular septal defect and patent ductus arteriosus are sufficiently characteristic to suggest the diagnosis within the first year of life. Noninvasive cardiac tests provide further clues to the diagnosis. Developments in echocardiography have revolutionized the diagnosis of congenital heart disease, permitting a definitive diagnosis of some of the more complex malformations without invasive testing. However, in many cases it is still necessary to resort to a combination of cardiac catheterization and angiocardiography.

Fetuses can be afflicted with a great variety of cardiac malformations, some of which cause stillbirth or death immediately after birth. Survivors' prognosis ranges from death in infancy to normal development and normal life span. The following discussion will present in detail six congenital lesions that account for more than 90 percent of congenital heart diseases permitting survival to adulthood (even without surgery).

Atrial Septal Defect

During fetal life communication between the two atria is essential for the fetus's survival. The foramen ovale, through which blood enters the left atrium, is protected by a valve that permits flow only from right to left. At birth, when pressure in the left side of the heart rises after the newborn takes its first breath, the foramen ovale ceases to function. Ordinarily it seals itself off, but even in cases when the sealing fails to occur, the valve does not permit it to func-

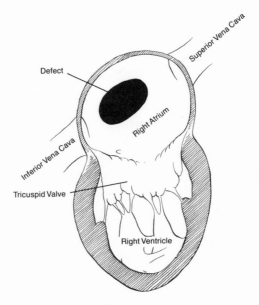

Figure 35. A typical atrial septal defect.

tion as a pathway for blood flow. Atrial septal defect is an abnormal opening, usually located in the region of the foramen ovale, but larger and wide-open, allowing large quantities of blood to flow from the left to the right atrium (fig. 35). The quantity of blood shunted through this communication varies according to the size of the defect and the capability of the right ventricle to accept the additional blood. Small atrial shunts have no serious effect on the circulation since left-to-right shunts do not reduce the oxygen content of the blood. Large shunts, however, can overload the right side of the heart and increase blood flow through the lungs as much as fourfold. Normally each heartbeat ejects from each ventricle into the respective arteries (aorta and pulmonary artery) an average of 75 cc of blood. In the case of a large atrial septal defect right ventricular ejection may increase to 300 cc, and left ventricular output remains normal; hence 225 cc of blood returns to the right side of the heart during systole. This is referred to as a four-to-one shunt (a ratio of pulmonary to systemic output). A large shunt not only overloads the right ventricle, producing its hypertrophy and dilatation, but the wear and tear on the small arteries in the lungs may damage their inner layer, which in some persons can lead to high pressure in the pulmonary arterial circulation. Pulmonary hypertension develops in about 15–20 percent of patients with atrial septal defect, almost always as adults. It may progress to the point where pressure in the right side of the heart exceeds that in the left, reversing the direction of blood flow from right to left through the shunt.

An atrial septal defect generally goes undetected until late childhood, adolescence, or even adulthood. The reason is that the flow through the defect between two low-pressure chambers does not produce turbulence audible as a murmur on physical examination. The child grows and develops normally (no cyanosis is present), except that the increased blood flow through the lungs raises susceptibility to respiratory infections. The diagnosis may be suggested on physical examination in older children by certain subtle abnormalities, but it is usually made when a chest X ray is taken, showing an enlarged heart and full blood vessels in the lungs. Confirmation of the diagnosis comes from echocardiography and cardiac catheterization, which reveals the magnitude of the shunt and the presence or absence of pulmonary vascular reaction (hypertension).

The course of atrial septal defect usually creates only minor problems. Development of the affected child is usually normal, although sometimes growth may be slightly impaired. Tolerance for exercise may be below average but seldom to the point of suggesting some disability. Frequent respiratory infections may occur. Persons in whom the defect is not surgically corrected may not develop significant symptoms until the fourth or fifth decade of life—sometimes even later. Reactive pulmonary hypertension, affecting one out of five patients with atrial septal defect, usually appears in early adulthood.

The treatment for atrial septal defect is surgical closure. This is one of the simplest cardiac operations, but it does require a pump-oxygenator. The operation is usually performed in older children or adolescents. Because of the risk of pulmonary hypertension it is best to close the defect before the age of 20. Closure of atrial septal defect is almost always a prophylactic operation performed on asymptomatic patients. If pulmonary hypertension is already present, closure may no longer be effective in preventing its progression. If cyanosis develops, closure of the defect is contraindicated since pulmonary hypertension then becomes the principal abnormality, which the operation will not correct.

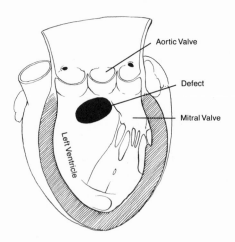

Figure 36. A typical ventricular septal defect.

Ventricular Septal Defect

Defect in the septum between the two ventricles is analogous to atrial septal defect in that it causes a unidirectional shunting of blood (fig. 36). An important difference between the two, however, makes ventricular septal defect a rather unique cardiac lesion. The two circulations, systemic and pulmonary, are closed systems: the former operates under high pressure determined by the resistance of small arteries, the latter under low pressure related to the minimal resistance of small branches of the pulmonary artery. Communication between the two circulations through the atria, where pressure in both chambers is close to zero, permits shunting of blood from one side to the other without significant consequences other than overload. However, communication between them in areas of high pressure—the ventricles or the arteries—may have disastrous consequences. A large opening between the two ventricles, with a systolic pressure of 120 mm Hg on the left side and 20 mm Hg on the right side produces a pressure gradient, so that most of the blood might escape to the right ventricle instead of entering the aorta. Clearly, a person could not survive were this allowed to happen; hence in compensation the systolic pressure in the right ventricle rises to match that in the left. Right ventricular systolic pressure can be elevated by one of two mechanisms—abnormal constriction of the small pulmonary arteries, increasing resistance to a level comparable to that of the systemic arteries and thereby producing pulmonary hypertension; or pulmonary valve stenosis.

A small ventricular septal defect is characterized by a left-to-right shunt through the opening because it offers enough resistance to blood flow to maintain the normal difference in pressures between the two ventricles. The magnitude of the shunt entirely depends on the size of the opening, which ranges from that of a pinhead to that of a dime. For the average adult heart the largest diameter consistent with a normal pressure relationship between the two ventricles is about 1.5 cm, the approximate dividing line between small and large ventricular septal defects. The blood flow through a ventricular septal defect produces turbulence and generates loud heart murmurs audible on examination of a child; hence the diagnosis of such a defect is usually made at birth or at least during infancy. The hemodynamic consequence of a small ventricular septal defect varies with the magnitude of the shunt. Small defects shunting no more than half of the left ventricular output into the right ventricle have no effect on circulatory dynamics. Although the heart murmur is still detectable, no other abnormalities are usually discovered. The prognosis is favorable, with a normal life expectancy. The only risk is the possibility of infective endocarditis. Surgical correction is usually considered unnecessary. A significant number of such patients experience spontaneous closure of the defect—in essence, self-cure. Larger shunts through small ventricular septal defects (greater than twice the left ventricular output) have effects similar to those of atrial septal defect, namely overload of the heart and overfilling of the pulmonary blood vessels. Since ventricular septal defect with large pulmonary flow but normal right ventricular pressure takes a similar course as atrial septal defect, surgical closure (by means of open-heart surgery) is generally performed in early childhood.

Large ventricular septal defect is a more serious problem. The normal function of the left ventricular pump has to be protected by pressure elevation in the right ventricle from birth; hence pulmonary hypertension is already present in infancy. The left-to-right shunting of blood is usually considerable. Persistent high pressure in the pulmonary arterial system, together with large blood flow in the pulmonary circulation, may gradually increase the resistance to the point of reversing the shunt from right to left. This complication happens occasionally in late childhood but most frequently in adulthood. Large ventricular septal defect complicated by shunt reversal and resulting in cyanosis is called *Eisenmenger's syndrome*. Despite pulmonary hypertension the growth and development of children with large ventricular septal defect are usually normal, and disability is rare. Even a fully developed cyanotic stage due to shunt reversal may be well tolerated, although in that case life expectancy is greatly reduced.

The treatment for large ventricular septal defect is surgical closure. The goal is to prevent progressive disease of small pulmonary arteries; thus surgical closure is often performed on small children, even infants. In the case of a large left-to-right shunt, closure of the defect may significantly reduce the pressure in the right ventricle and lower or even eliminate pulmonary hypertension. Large ventricular septal defect also occurs in combination with pulmonary stenosis, in which case pulmonary hypertension is absent (see discussion of tetralogy of Fallot below).

Patent Ductus Arteriosus

During the fetal period the ductus arteriosus connecting the descending aorta with the pulmonary artery serves as an essential pathway supplying blood partly oxygenated by the placenta to the arteries of the lower part of the fetal body. Normally the duct closes immediately after birth, but owing to a developmental error it may remain open, or *patent*, in some infants. The altered pressure conditions during postnatal life (higher in the systemic circulation than in the pulmonary circulation) allows blood to flow through the duct in the opposite direction, that is, from the aorta to the pulmonary artery. This left-to-right shunt on the arterial level is analogous to the atrial and ventricular septal defects. As in the other two conditions, fully oxygenated blood returns to the lungs; gas exchange proceeds normally, but the excess blood may overfill the pulmonary circulation. Since that excess has to be pumped into the aorta by the left ventricle, the latter may be affected by the increased workload if the shunt volume is large.

The size of persistent ducts varies widely. A small duct has no significant effect on circulatory dynamics but is at risk of developing infective endarteritis (an infection analogous to endocarditis, striking the arteries rather than the heart). The turbulent flow through the duct produces an audible murmur in the patient's chest different from murmurs caused by lesions inside the heart. A large duct, by overloading the left ventricle and the pulmonary circulation, may produce pulmonary hypertension in adulthood. Rarely, a very large duct shunts so much blood away from the aorta of an infant that a surgical emergency is created.

Surgical correction of patent ductus arteriosus consists of tying off the duct in an operation that does not require use of the pump-oxygenator. The duct can also sometimes be closed through a non-surgical technique involving cardiac catheterization. The simplicity and low risk of duct closure justifies its performance even in cases where the condition has no effect on the circulation, to guard against infection. Spontaneous closure of the duct occurs in infancy or childhood in an estimated 5 percent of cases.

Pulmonary Stenosis

Congenital stenosis of the outflow segment of the right ventricle may be a sole malformation or part of a complex combination of defects. The simplest variety of pulmonary stenosis is fusion of the three leaflets of the pulmonary valve into a single membranelike structure with an opening in the center. As in other forms of valvular stenosis, the size of the opening directly determines its effect on circulatory dynamics. Pulmonary stenosis, if significant, places a pressure overload on the right ventricle analogous to the effect of aortic stenosis on the left ventricle (see chap. 9). The resistance to outflow from the right ventricle elevates the pressure inside that chamber, causing a pressure gradient between the ventricle and the pulmonary artery, where the pressure remains normal. In health identical pressures in the right ventricle and the pulmonary artery in systole average 15 mm Hg. In mild pulmonary stenosis right ventricular systolic pressure may rise to about 40 mm Hg; in moderate, to 70 mm Hg; and in severe, to 150 mm Hg. The right ventricle is quite able to adapt to the high pressure, particularly in infancy. However, in severe pulmonary stenosis the overloaded right ventricle may eventually produce right ventricular failure. In rare cases severe pulmonary stenosis may lead to serious emergencies in infancy requiring immediate surgical intervention.

Mild cases of pulmonary stenosis require no treatment other than preventive measures against endocarditis. Severe pulmonary stenosis requires surgical relief. Pulmonary valvotomy by means of open-heart surgery was the standard treatment until the late 1980s. Balloon dilatation of the pulmonary valve has now been applied successfully and is becoming the treatment of choice. The use of prosthetic valves in pulmonary stenosis is rarely necessary.

Tetralogy of Fallot

Tetralogy of Fallot represents a combination of pulmonary stenosis and large ventricular septal defect. It is the most important malformation associated with persistent cyanosis, the commonest cause of "blue baby." The term "tetralogy" was suggested more than a century ago, when two other features (making a total of four) were considered central to this malformation. These two features are now known to be consequences of the first two.

The most essential component of this lesion is large ventricular septal defect. The obligatory high pressure in the right ventricle is, however, maintained by pulmonary stenosis rather than by high resistance in the pulmonary circulation, as is the case in isolated ventricular septal defect. The narrowing may be located either at the valve or below the valve (*subvalvular pulmonary stenosis*). In some cases not only is the valve or the outflow segment of the right ventricle affected by the malformation, but the pulmonary artery may be smaller than average (*hypoplastic*), compounding the difficulty in the pulmonary circulation. In most cases the resistance to outflow from the right ventricle is higher than that from the left ventricle—hence the reversal of blood flow (right-to-left shunt) resulting in cyanosis. When pulmonary stenosis is relatively mild, the usual left-to-right shunt through the ventricular septal defect takes place (noncyanotic tetralogy of Fallot). The wide variation in the resistances within the pulmonary outflow tract creates a range of skin coloration in children with tetralogy of Fallot—some showing normal color, others a faintly blue tinge, still others a deep purple color. In black children and other children with naturally dark skin, the effects of cyanosis may be less apparent. Despite the complexity of this malformation of the heart, survival beyond infancy is possible in most cases; development may be mildly impaired, but many patients reach adulthood, some even surviving beyond middle age.

One of the most spectacular advances in treating congenital heart disease was the operation introduced in 1944 by Alfred Blalock and Helen Taussig. This procedure crafted a connection between the systemic circulation and the pulmonary circulation by suturing the large artery supplying the arm (brachial artery) into the pulmonary artery branch; the arterial blood, poorly oxygenated because of mixing with venous blood through the right-to-left shunt, could thereby return to the lungs for reoxygenation. The drama of deeply blue children assuming a pink color after the operation created a sensation when it was first performed. This operation is now rarely used since it does not attack the basic defect. Open-heart surgery allows surgeons to close the ventricular septal defect and dilate the right ventricular outflow tract; the procedure is performed on patients in infancy or early childhood.

Coarctation of the Aorta

It is customary to include in any discussion of congenital heart disease *coarctation of the aorta,* even though it is a vascular, not a cardiac, malformation. It involves a congenital narrowing of the aorta in the region where the aortic arch changes into the descending aorta. This stenosis is usually severe, bordering on complete interruption of flow into the descending aorta. The flow of arterial blood into the head and upper extremities is unimpaired, but the rest of the body has to receive blood via a detour—collateral circulation. Branches of the aorta supplying blood to the upper part of the body form connections with branches of the descending aorta, especially arteries supplying the chest that run between the ribs. These connections function so that when some of the arterial blood meant for the upper parts of the body reaches the arteries in the chest, it flows in the opposite direction, into the descending aorta. As a consequence of the abnormally high resistance caused by redirection of the blood, patients usually suffer from high blood pressure, which may overload the left ventricle and cause its hypertrophy.

Coarctation of the aorta accounts for many cases of high blood pressure in infants, children, and adolescents. Such hypertension is curable, disappearing when the coarctation is corrected. Although hypertension is the most serious consequence of coarctation, rare complications include infective endarteritis, stroke caused by small aneurysms of an artery supplying the brain, and aortic dissection (see chap. 14).

Other Congenital
Malformations of the Heart

Transposition of the great arteries is a complex but common malformation. Before surgical procedures allowing partial or total correction were developed, few afflicted with this defect survived childhood. With surgical treatment patients may now reach adulthood, though their life expectancy remains greatly reduced. This malformation consists of an error in cardiac development wherein the aorta arises from the right ventricle and the pulmonary artery from the left (fig. 37). The transposition creates two separate closed circulations incapable of the exchange of gases in the blood necessary for survival: deoxygenated blood returning to the right heart through systemic veins is ejected into the aorta without being able to acquire oxygen and dispose of carbon dioxide. Blood returning fully oxygenated from the lungs enters the pulmonary artery and returns to the lungs. Obviously, this situation is incompatible with survival unless some mixing of the two bloods takes place. That need is met by persistence in the infant of the fetal communication between the two circulations, namely the foramen ovale. Occasionally ventricular septal defect is also present and assists in the mixing. Infants surviving on this oxygen-poor blood have a dark purple coloration of the skin; if a sizable proportion of the oxygenated blood is shunted into the arterial side, survival beyond infancy is possible without operation. Several methods of correcting the defect are now available, restoring normal color and permitting survival into adulthood.

Pulmonary atresia consists of total closure of the outlet for blood from the right ventricle. All the venous blood returning to the right side of the heart is shunted to the left side through atrial and sometimes ventricular septal defects. The fully mixed blood reaches the pulmonary artery and the lungs via a patent ductus arteriosus. Deep cyanosis is usually present.

Tricuspid atresia involves an absence of communication between

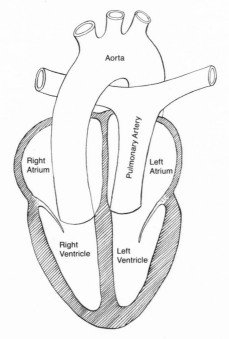

Figure 37. The circulation in complete
transposition of the great vessels.
Communication between the two sides of the
heart, necessary for survival, is not shown in the
drawing.

the right atrium and the right ventricle. Venous blood is shunted
through a defect into the left atrium, and the mixed blood enters
the lungs through the ductus arteriosus.

Total anomalous venous return consists of malposition of the
pulmonary veins carrying oxygenated blood, which enter the right
atrium instead of the left atrium, resulting in total mixing of unoxygenated and oxygenated blood. The mixture is shunted through an
atrial septal defect into the left atrium and is ejected by the left
ventricle in the aorta.

Ebstein's anomaly involves malposition of the tricuspid valve
well inside the right ventricle, reducing its capacity. The foramen
ovale often remains patent, allowing a portion of the blood from the
right atrium to be shunted to the left side. The extent of cyanosis
varies according to the size of the right-to-left shunt through the

foramen ovale. This lesion permits survival to adulthood and occasionally to old age.

Truncus arteriosus is a malformation of the great arteries attached to the heart. A single artery is connected with both ventricles, which communicate through a ventricular septal defect. This arterial trunk divides into a pulmonary artery and aorta. Total mixing of the blood occurs in the trunk.

Single ventricle occurs when the entire septum between the two ventricles is absent. This malformation produces complete mixing of oxygenated and unoxygenated blood.

These seven malformations have in common the mixing of oxygenated and unoxygenated blood in the systemic arteries. As a consequence, the tissues receive blood poorer in oxygen than is normal. Survivors are capable of growth, development, and some activity. Surgical treatment is now available for most of these syndromes, with variable results.

Congenital malformations without shunting of blood involve abnormalities of cardiac valves. Pulmonary stenosis has already been discussed in this chapter; left-sided cardiac valvular diseases are presented in chapter 9. Aortic stenosis is a relatively common congenital malformation, mostly as a valvular stenosis involving fusion of the three leaflets of the aortic valve. Rare variants of stenosis of the left-sided outflow segment of the ventricle include *subvalvular stenosis,* in which a membrane with a central opening stretches across the outflow segment underneath a normal aortic valve, and *supravalvular stenosis,* a narrowing of the aorta just above the aortic valve. A common anomaly of the aortic valve is the *bicuspid valve* (two leaflets instead of three), which has no effect on the heart and circulation but may be the site for deposition of calcium late in life and hence a cause of calcific aortic stenosis. Congenital mitral stenosis is rare as an isolated malformation, although it is seen in combination with other defects.

Chapter Twelve

Hypertension

Normal arterial blood pressure shows wide variation. The systolic pressure ranges from 100 to 140 mm Hg, and the diastolic pressure from 60 to 90 mm Hg. These upper and lower limits are derived from measurements of a large sampling of healthy persons. They cannot, however, be considered sharp cutoff points separating the healthy from those suffering from *hypertension* ("high blood pressure") or *hypotension* ("low blood pressure"). Hypertension is considered significant only if persistent and repeated readings of blood pressure above the norm, generally much higher than the maximum levels, are discovered. Both abnormally high and abnormally low blood pressure are clinical findings, not in themselves a disease. Abnormally elevated blood pressure occurs under certain circumstances in healthy persons; it can be a manifestation of disease elsewhere in the body *(secondary hypertension)*. But if persistent, it indicates primary disease. It is this primary disease *(essential hypertension)* that is the principal subject of this chapter.

Disturbances of Regulation of Blood Pressure

The regulatory mechanism for maintaining blood pressure at a constant level was presented in chapter 2. This barostatic mechanism (similar to temperature regulation by thermostats) is capable of regulating resistance to blood flow by opening and closing the arterioles to compensate for variation in cardiac output. This pressure regulatory center is located at the base of the brain, where it receives and sends out signals via the autonomic nervous system. However, the response of the arterioles to these impulses can be either strengthened or weakened by chemical substances circulating in the blood. Thus disturbances of pressure regulation can be related to one of two mechanisms: either the barostatic center is set too high or too low, so that improper nervous impulses reach the arterioles (*neurogenic mechanism*), or normal nervous impulses are improperly modified by the presence of chemical substances (*humoral mechanism*). Chemical substances that raise blood pressure by sensitizing arteriolar responses to nervous impulses are called *pressor* substances; those that desensitize responses and lower blood pressure are called *depressor* substances. Such pressor and depressor effects are the properties of many chemical substances—hormones normally produced in the body, hormones produced only under abnormal conditions, and drugs.

Disturbances of either the neurogenic or humoral mechanism may occur temporarily or permanently. For example, blood pressure may rise in healthy persons during periods of stress, anger, and excitement, presumably because of an excess of normal pressor hormones. Conversely, temporary falls in blood pressure may result from prolonged standing (fatigue of regulatory center), causing fainting. Furthermore, regulation of blood pressure may be imperfect, leading to abnormal drops in blood pressure when the person switches from a lying to a standing position (*postural hypotension*). Permanent disturbances of blood pressure—hypertension or hypotension—may be caused secondarily by disturbances of other organs; however, only hypertension can be a primary, potentially serious disease. Hypotension is consistent with good health and is most frequently merely a variant of the norm, although occasionally it may be a sign of some systemic disease (long-standing wasting diseases such as cancer, tuberculosis, or Addison's disease).

The kidneys play an important role in the regulation of blood pressure. Special cells in the kidneys secrete *renin*, a chemical that combines with a protein circulating in the blood to produce *angiotensin I*. This compound has no significant effect on the circulation but is rapidly changed by an enzyme into *angiotensin II*, a powerful pressor hormone essential in regulating blood pressure. Furthermore, angiotensin II is the principal factor stimulating the adrenal cortex to secrete *aldosterone,* which regulates salt and water content in the body. This reaction is referred to as the renin-angiotensin-aldosterone axis. Excess formation of renin may initiate the process leading to hypertension; furthermore, ingestion of salt (sodium) in the diet facilitates the development of hypertension, whereas significant reduction of salt intake lowers blood pressure. The renin mechanism is directly involved in one type of secondary hypertension (renovascular hypertension) and may be implicated in some cases of essential hypertension.

The relationship between the kidneys and hypertension has been known since blood pressure measurements first became available at the turn of the century; in the 1930s high blood pressure was experimentally produced in an animal by interfering with the blood supply to the kidneys, thereby stimulating excessive production of renin. Stenosis of the renal artery (supplying the kidney) was experimentally induced, causing hypertension in the animal; relief of the stenosis brought the blood pressure back to normal.

Causes of Hypertension

Most patients with high blood pressure have essential hypertension (sometimes referred to as "idiopathic," since its cause is unknown). It accounts for about 95 percent of all cases of hypertension. Many patients with essential hypertension show increased activity of renin in the blood. This finding led to the hypothesis that disturbance of the renin-angiotensin-aldosterone axis is the cause of essential hypertension as well as of hypertension due to demonstrable abnormalities of renal blood supply. However, excess of these hormones could not be demonstrated consistently in patients with hypertension; thus the hypothesis has not been confirmed, although the renin mechanism plays a contributory role in many patients. There is some controversy as to whether hypertensive patients with high renin activity represent a subgroup with a different course and prognosis than those with low or normal renin activity. One feature of essential hypertension generally accepted, however, is its tendency to run in families, which indicates a hereditary factor.

Secondary hypertension (5 percent of all cases of hypertension) may occur in the course of many diseases. Some diseases of the kidneys produce elevated blood pressure (*renal hypertension*), though there is no definite relationship between impaired kidney function and hypertension. These include acute glomerulonephritis, chronic nephritis, pylonephritis, and polycystic kidney disease. Renovascular hypertension includes demonstrable abnormalities in the arterial blood supply to the kidney. Renal and renovascular hypertension account for about 80 percent of the cases of secondary hypertension. *Endocrine hypertension* is caused by tumors secreting an excess of hormones involved in pressure regulation or by abnormally increased hormone production in hyperactive glands. This category includes *pheochromocytoma*, a tumor secreting epinephrine or norepinephrine (normal hormones of the medulla of the adrenal glands); *primary aldosteronism*, an excess of the hormone of the adrenal cortex; and *Cushing's syndrome*, or hyperplasia of the pituitary gland. Hypertension may also be a secondary effect of coarctation of the aorta (see chap. 11), excess female hormones (such as in the abnormal reaction of some women to contraceptive pills and hypertension developing during pregnancy), and some disturbances of the central nervous system.

Consequences and Course
of Hypertension

Hypertension is not a well-defined disease but rather a nonspecific circulatory abnormality. It can be produced by several different mechanisms, and if it lasts long enough, it can be disabling or even shorten life. The characteristic feature of hypertension is that it does not produce symptoms in the vast majority of patients, who may remain unaware of any problem even when serious consequences of hypertension are already present. Some of the symptoms traditionally ascribed to hypertension, such as headache or dizziness, are relatively rare, and their relationship to elevated blood pressure is uncertain.

The question of when blood pressure should be considered abnormally high is still subject to debate. The accepted criterion in the United States is that normal pressure should not exceed 140 mm Hg systolic and 90 mm Hg diastolic. The World Health Organization accepts as normal blood pressure readings up to 160/95. The difficulty in diagnosing hypertension is compounded by the wide variability of blood pressure in healthy persons; hence a single blood pressure reading is not a reliable basis for diagnosis. Normal variations are related to many factors, including responses to stimuli—stress, exercise, fear, or excitement. Physicians have long recognized that the blood pressure reading in a patient seen in the office for the first time is usually higher than subsequent readings, and the difference may be considerable. Some people always tense up in the doctor's office and show abnormally high blood pressure, although at other times their pressure may be normal; in the medical literature this condition is sometimes referred to as "white coat hypertension."

Proper diagnosis of hypertension must be based on repeated findings of abnormally high blood pressure. Often patients are taught to take their own blood pressure and are instructed to keep charts with periodic readings of blood pressure over several days. Portable automatic blood pressure monitors are also available; the patient wears the monitor for 12 or more hours, during which time frequent readings are registered.

Observations in patients with long-standing hypertension have revealed that the diastolic pressure is less variable than the systolic pressure. Hence the severity of hypertension is customarily classified according to diastolic pressure:

mild hypertension—90–104 mm Hg

moderate hypertension—105–119 mm Hg

severe hypertension—greater than 120 mm Hg

These levels represent averages of repeated readings rather than an isolated reading. One of the difficulties in evaluating the severity of hypertension is that many patients have unusually variable blood pressure, with grossly abnormal "overshoots" as well as normal pressures appearing periodically. Such patients are thought to have "labile," or unstable, hypertension, and the need for treatment has to be individually evaluated. Although variable, the systolic pressure level is closely related to the long-term consequences of hypertension.

Drug therapy for hypertension is relatively recent. The first drugs became available in the 1950s, but the full effect of successful therapy is much more recent than that. To comprehend the dramatic effects of drug therapy, we need only review the course and prognosis of untreated hypertension before antihypertensive therapy was widely available. The principal consequences of severe hypertension for the cardiovascular system include the following:

increased workload on the left ventricle of the heart, producing its
  hypertrophy and eventual failure

acceleration of atherosclerotic damage to various organs due to the
  wear and tear of high pressure on the arteries

kidney damage, leading to kidney failure (uremia)

damage to the retina of the eye, leading to disturbances of vision

brain damage (stroke), including hemorrhage (often fatal)

complications directly related to high pressures in the arterial system, including aortic dissection (partial rupture of the aorta) and rupture of weakened areas in the arteries of the brain ("berry aneurysm," a small blisterlike outpouching of the wall of an artery), causing cerebral hemorrhage

The effect of hypertension on the heart is its commonest and most serious sequel. Left ventricular hypertrophy leads to heart failure, to accelerated coronary atherosclerosis, and to the risk of sudden death from arrhythmia. Atherosclerosis related to hypertension may also produce stroke and serious disabling disease of the arteries of the legs.

Hypertension induces damage to the small arteries of the kidneys (*nephrosclerosis*), which may interfere with the principal function of the kidneys—excretion of waste products in the urine. The effect of hypertension on the retinal arteries in the back of the eye is of diagnostic importance since these small vessels are visible through an ophthalmoscope. Early changes produced by hypertension can be detected before any other consequences of high blood pressure are discovered. The severity of damage to the eye is classified according to the magnitude of detected abnormalities. However, vision is only affected in the last stage, when there is swelling in the critical portion of the eye (*papilledema*).

Untreated essential hypertension typically progresses at a very slow pace, so that the consequent damage takes many years to develop. It is often referred to as "benign hypertension," to distinguish it from a small subgroup of hypertension that progresses rapidly, "malignant hypertension." (If existing benign hypertension suddenly accelerates, the condition is called the "malignant phase.") Malignant hypertension may develop as a variant of either essential hypertension or some types of secondary hypertension. It is characterized by high blood pressure, particularly diastolic pressure, which may rise to 130–150 mm Hg. Severe damage to eye vessels affecting vision is common, as is kidney failure, in addition to its cardiac consequences. Some of these changes are irreversible, although aggressive therapy is capable of reversing and controlling malignant hypertension.

A rare complication of hypertension, most often found in malignant cases, is a hypertensive crisis, an acute event usually manifested as *hypertensive encephalopathy.* It is a life-threatening emergency consisting of an acute rise of blood pressure producing malfunction of the brain—confusion, loss of consciousness, and convulsions. When this complication develops in women afflicted with hypertension during pregnancy, it is known as *eclampsia.* Prompt aggressive therapy usually relieves the crisis and reverses its manifestations. Other complications of hypertension producing emergencies include acute pulmonary edema, myocardial infarction, and aortic dissection.

Untreated severe hypertension, though still encountered, is now uncommon, although milder degrees are very frequent in the general population, especially older people. The course of hypertension as it is seen today is entirely different because of effective drug therapy. Wide dissemination of knowledge regarding the importance of early treatment of high blood pressure has completely altered the course and natural history of hypertension. Yet since hypertension produces practically no symptoms, people occasionally carry this disease for a long time without being aware of it. Furthermore, some patients may neglect prescribed treatment, which requires some motivation and cooperation. But even poorly designed or sporadically pursued treatment exerts some effect by protecting against the most serious effects of this disease. Today poorly controlled hypertension is principally recognized as a risk factor in atherosclerosis, thus increasing the probability of myocardial infarction, stroke, and other atherosclerotic diseases.

Treatment of Hypertension

One of the more difficult decisions in medicine is how to treat hypertension. Though a potentially life-threatening—certainly a life-shortening—disease, in most patients hypertension is consistent with good general health. Yet a diagnosis of hypertension may require a commitment on the part of the patient to lifelong use of one or more drugs that frequently produce undesirable side effects—to put it bluntly, may make a well person sick. Consequently, before the initiation of antihypertensive therapy some questions need to be considered. Can the patient safely be left untreated? Could nonpharmacological treatment be effective? Could the patient have one of the rare curable varieties of hypertension that can be eliminated by a surgical intervention?

Differentiating between normal variations in blood pressure with unusual overshoots and true hypertension is difficult. This fact, together with observations showing that serious consequences of hypertension are mostly found in severe hypertension, has led to a controversy regarding the treatment of mild hypertension (diastolic pressure averaging less than 105 mm Hg). Some experts recommend treatment even in the mildest cases of hypertension; others favor postponing therapy, while maintaining careful supervision, unless the patient enters the stage of moderate hypertension. More often, however, early treatment of mild hypertension is advised. Antihypertensive therapy is tailored to each patient according to the degree of hypertension and the patient's motivation in adhering strictly to instructions involved in drug therapy.

Before starting therapy, the patient undergoes a careful evaluation to determine the extent of damage to body organs from the existing hypertension. If an abnormal electrocardiogram or echocardiogram demonstrates left ventricular hypertrophy, abnormalities of the vessels in the eye or impaired kidney function, aggressive therapy is mandatory, even if hypertension is only mild at the time of discovery. In cases of mild hypertension nonpharmacological therapy is tried first; such treatment is most successful in this group of patients. It includes reducing sodium (salt) in the diet, reducing body weight if the patient is overweight, avoiding stressful situations, engaging in recreational activities, and establishing a regular exercise program.

Only 2 percent of the cases of hypertension are curable. Certain screening tests may suggest such a possibility and justify more-elaborate studies. The search for reversible secondary hypertension is usually limited to cases in which unusual findings are present, such as severe or rapidly progressive hypertension in young persons; in addition, certain syndromes atypical of essential hypertension may point to some underlying disease responsible for the hypertension.

Most patients treated for hypertension are apparently healthy and asymptomatic persons with mild or moderate hypertension who are committed to prolonged drug therapy. Since the introduction of effective antihypertensive drugs in the 1950s, nearly 50 different drugs have been approved for treatment of hypertension, and the number of new drugs is constantly increasing.

Drugs are classified according to their effect on a specific function involved in regulating blood pressure. Most drugs in each class have similar—often identical—action and can be used interchangeably, although manufacturers often claim the superiority of one drug over the others. The important categories of antihypertensive drugs are

diuretics, which enhance salt excretion

drugs reducing or blocking vascular control exerted by the sympathetic nervous system

drugs dilating arterioles and thereby reducing resistance (and pressure)

drugs blocking the flow of calcium into cells

drugs inhibiting the angiotensin-converting enzyme

Antihypertensive therapy demands collaboration between physician and patient. To begin, one of the "first-line" antihypertensive agents least likely to have side effects is usually administered and the dose adjusted according to its effectiveness. Undesirable side effects may require switching to a drug from another class. Large doses of a single drug are often avoided in favor of adding a second drug. In severe hypertension or drug-resistant hypertension it may be necessary to use a combination of several drugs. Success in such therapy is gauged by the patient's tolerance for drugs and the effective reduction of blood pressure. Patients who tolerate drugs poorly may have to settle for more-modest therapeutic goals, such as reducing moderate or severe hypertension to mild hypertension. Whereas in most cases effective and well-tolerated drugs can be found easily, in drug-resistant patients a prolonged period of drug testing by trial and error may be necessary.

Chapter Thirteen

Diseases of the Pulmonary Circulation

The lesser, or pulmonary, circulation differs in many respects from the systemic circulation. The volume of blood directed into a single organ, the lungs, equals that ejected into the aorta for the entire remainder of the body. Pressure in the pulmonary circulation is influenced by many factors, in contrast to pressure in the systemic circulation, which is controlled solely by constriction and relaxation of the arterioles. The arterial pressure in the pulmonary circulation is roughly one-fifth that in the systemic circulation. With these differences it is not surprising that abnormalities affecting the pulmonary circulation are unlike those affecting other regions of the circulation.

The principal significance of disturbances of the pulmonary circulation is that they impose an increased workload on the right ventricle of the heart, which may produce its hypertrophy and failure. (Similar effects on the left side of the heart result from problems of the systemic circulation, as we have seen.) Such overload within this circuit is caused primarily by two mechanisms: increased blood flow to the lungs and increased pressure within the pulmonary circulation. Increased blood flow is a characteristic feature of left-to-right shunts, occurring almost exclusively in congenital heart disease (see chapter 11). Pulmonary hypertension is the primary problem in disorders of the pulmonary circulation. It is of such magnitude and complexity that it will be presented here in its entirety at the risk of repeating some points already made in previous chapters.

Pulmonary Hypertension

Knowledge concerning pulmonary hypertension is relatively new. In contrast to the systemic arterial pressure, which can be measured by a simple apparatus, the sphygmomanometer, pressures within the pulmonary circulation can only be measured during cardiac catheterization or indirectly by Doppler echocardiography. Consequently, a major procedure must be performed each time pressure in the pulmonary artery has to be obtained. Elevated pressure in the pulmonary artery can be caused by one of three principal mechanisms: (1) increased resistance within the pulmonary vascular tree, (2) increased blood flow through the lungs, and (3) increased pressure in the left atrium transmitted back through the pulmonary veins into the pulmonary arterial system.

Pulmonary hypertension owing to increased resistance within the pulmonary circulation may be caused by several factors. Spasm and constriction of the pulmonary arterioles—the only mechanism within the pulmonary circulation analogous to mechanisms of systemic hypertension—occur in a variety of diseases. Great efforts are being made to reveal the circumstances under which pulmonary arterial spasm may be successfully eliminated, restoring more-normal pressure in the pulmonary circulation. Other factors causing increased resistance include organic changes within the arterial tree, closing off some channels; occlusion of smaller branches of the pulmonary artery by emboli; and the sudden blockage of the main pulmonary artery or its principal branches by a large thrombus.

Pulmonary arteriolar spasm leading to pulmonary hypertension may be caused by specific stimuli. Two such stimuli have been discovered, and their role in pulmonary hypertension is considerable: (1) reduced oxygen content in the blood (*hypoxemia*), such as occurs at high altitude or in some diseases of the lungs, and (2) increased pressure within the left atrium, characteristic of mitral stenosis and left ventricular failure. Pulmonary arteriolar spasm caused by these stimuli is reversible, and their elimination produces a fall in pulmonary arterial pressure.

Pulmonary hypertension caused by increased blood flow to the lungs is almost entirely restricted to congenital heart disease. An increase in blood flow within the pulmonary circulation does not automatically raise pressure within this circuit. The lungs have a large vascular reserve capacity that can accommodate excess blood without increasing resistance to flow. Thus in healthy persons during exercise cardiac output increases without raising pressure in the pulmonary circulation. Large shunts due to the various congenital communications between the two sides of the circulation may persist without elevating pressure in the pulmonary circuit. However, for various reasons the reserve capacity of the pulmonary vascular tree may not be available in some cases of congenital heart disease, so that pulmonary arterial pressure rises in direct proportion to increases of pulmonary blood flow. This type of pulmonary hypertension associated with congenital heart disease is called *hyperkinetic pulmonary hypertension.*

Pressure transmitted backward from the left atrium is termed *passive pulmonary hypertension.* High left atrial pressure in mitral stenosis and in left ventricular failure dams up the blood flow and forces the right ventricle to eject blood under high pressure. This passive pulmonary hypertension is not to be confused with pulmonary arteriolar spasm, which is also related to rise in pressure in the left atrium and can occur in conjunction with passive elevation of pressure.

Pulmonary hypertension presents problems to the physician different from those related to systemic arterial hypertension. The latter, in addition to causing overload of the left ventricle, may have such secondary serious effects as accelerating atherosclerotic disease of the coronary circulation and other regions and damaging the kidneys and brain. Such secondary effects do not develop in pulmonary hypertension, and its problems concern primarily its effects on the right ventricle. However, the challenge of pulmonary hypertension is that it occurs frequently in children and young adults and produces significant disability earlier than does systemic hypertension. The crucial question involving pulmonary hypertension is its reversibility. Some forms respond well to treatment of their causes. Surgical closure of a left-to-right shunt associated with hyperkinetic pulmonary hypertension brings about an immediate fall in pulmonary arterial pressure, which can be measured during surgery. Similarly, in passive pulmonary hypertension relief of mitral stenosis producing a fall in left atrial pressure immediately lowers pulmonary pressure. Other forms of reversible pulmonary hypertension are less dramatic and may require more time for a fall in pressure. These include pulmonary arteriolar spasm related to high left atrial pressure and hypoxemia.

Perhaps the most striking point about pulmonary hypertension is that certain reversible varieties turn into permanent and irreversible forms. This transition occurs most frequently in congenital heart disease associated with high pulmonary blood flow and is related to the development of organic diseases of the small pulmonary blood vessels. The importance of this self-perpetuating form of pulmonary hypertension has been discussed in connection with ventricular septal defect and other forms of congenital disease (chapter 11). Since in congenital heart disease pulmonary hypertension is the leading factor in reducing the lifespan of children and young adults, the physician has to be acutely aware that a patient may at one point have a reversible form of pulmonary hypertension and be a candidate for complete surgical cure but a year or two later, if surgical treatment is postponed, may develop an inoperable form because of pulmonary vascular disease.

Diseases Affecting the
Pulmonary Circulation
Pulmonary Embolism

Perhaps the most serious and unpredictable condition affecting the pulmonary circulation is pulmonary embolism. It consists of occlusion of sections of the pulmonary arterial tree by thrombi carried in the bloodstream from the venous part of the circulation or from the right side of the heart. The sites of formation of thrombi vary. Whereas inflammatory diseases of the veins are usually associated with thrombosis (thrombophlebitis), pulmonary embolism occurs much more frequently in veins not affected by inflammation (phlebothrombosis). It is known that in susceptible persons thrombi can form in veins, particularly during periods of inactivity. The veins most commonly affected by "silent" thrombosis are deep veins of the legs (not varicose veins) and veins in the pelvic organs (reproductive organs in women and the prostate in men). Because inactivity is an important cause of such thrombi, venous thrombosis and pulmonary emboli are particularly likely to develop in people who are bedridden.

Several types of pulmonary embolism can be distinguished. In *pulmonary infarct* a small single embolus affects a small segment of a lung, which becomes clogged with blood. This relatively benign condition may cause chest pain, spitting up of blood, and some fever; it appears on the chest X ray as a shadow similar to that of pneumonia. Prompt recovery usually occurs in a single infarct without sequelae. The significance of pulmonary infarct is as a predictor of larger, more serious emboli developing from the source of the small embolus.

A large pulmonary embolism or multiple emboli can cause overloading of the pulmonary circulation. When a certain area of the pulmonary arterial tree (usually more than half) is occluded by clots, pressure in the pulmonary artery rises. The sudden onset of pulmonary hypertension often does not give the heart time to adapt and rapidly leads to right ventricular failure. Such an event, occasionally referred to as acute cor pulmonale, can be fatal, but it may reverse itself when pulmonary emboli are no longer forthcoming, either because of cessation of thrombosis or in response to surgical intervention. Patients with acute cor pulmonale are short of breath, may be in shock, and show signs of right ventricular failure.

Massive pulmonary embolism occluding the main pulmonary artery or the two principal branches causes death, usually instantly and without warning. It is the prevention of this dreaded complication that has placed so much emphasis on signs of any disturbance of the venous circulation.

Small, repeated pulmonary emboli may feed the pulmonary circulation over a period of weeks, months, or years, causing gradual elevation of pressure in the pulmonary artery and leading to chronic, irreversible pulmonary hypertension. Fortunately uncommon, this severe, usually fatal form of pulmonary hypertension is almost indistinguishable from primary pulmonary hypertension.

Treatment of pulmonary embolism mainly involves anticoagulant therapy to prevent recurrences of emboli. Acute cases may call for thrombolytic therapy. Interventional therapy includes surgical removal of clots, located by angiography, from the pulmonary artery or its principal branches. Various methods of occluding the inferior vena cava in cases where emboli are thought to arise in the lower part of the body are occasionally used. Occlusion blocks the pathway for emboli and forces the blood to return to the heart through small collateral veins.

Cor Pulmonale

The term "cor pulmonale" literally means heart disease related to the lungs or pulmonary circulation; it should logically include all disturbances of the pulmonary circulation. However, in current medical terminology the term "chronic cor pulmonale" is used exclusively to indicate the cardiac effect of chronic diseases of the lungs. "Acute cor pulmonale" has already been mentioned as referring to large pulmonary embolism, but there are some who question any use of the term "cor pulmonale" not connected with diseases of the lungs.

The essential feature of chronic cor pulmonale is pulmonary hypertension caused most frequently by hypoxemia. Thus cor pulmonale occurs when some parts of the lungs remain unventilated, though their blood supply is unimpaired, as in the late stages of pulmonary emphysema, pulmonary fibrosis, and some varieties of chronic bronchitis. Other, rarer conditions producing chronic hypoxemia include chronic mountain sickness (an exaggerated response in some persons to low oxygen content at high altitude) and extreme obesity. These two conditions are of course reversible—chronic mountain sickness by transferring the patient to a location at sea level, obesity by dieting. As a rule, however, chronic cor pulmonale is a serious condition indicating the late stages of lung disease. Treatment is limited to controlling heart failure and is usually ineffective.

Primary Pulmonary Hypertension

A rare, severe disease, primary pulmonary hypertension usually affects young adults and occasionally children; its cause is unknown. The onset of the disease is inconspicuous and its progress very slow, causing excessive fatigue and shortness of breath. Patients may live for several years partly incapacitated, but they eventually develop intractable heart failure. Treatment has little to offer: various drugs used for essential hypertension have been tried, but success, if any, is only of short duration. In cases where there is even a suspicion that pulmonary hypertension may have been caused by repeated small emboli, anticoagulant therapy may arrest the progress of the disease, though significant improvement is uncommon.

Other Diseases Associated with Pulmonary Hypertension

The conditions discussed above cause pulmonary hypertension, which is their primary link with heart disease. There are a number of diseases of the heart in which pulmonary hypertension develops secondarily and is only one of several factors affecting the heart. They include congenital heart disease, mitral stenosis and mitral insufficiency, and chronic failure of the left ventricle of the heart. These conditions may produce all three types of pulmonary hypertension—passive, hyperkinetic, and that related to high pulmonary vascular resistance. However, the first two types are less likely to cause severe pulmonary hypertension than the third. Consequently, in ordinary clinical terms the phrase "pulmonary hypertension" is most often applied to elevated pulmonary vascular resistance. Thus pulmonary hypertension in connection with mitral stenosis connotes that in addition to passive elevation of pressure in the pulmonary artery, arteriolar constriction has taken place. In congenital heart disease, separating operable cases with high flow (hyperkinetic) from inoperable cases with high resistance constitutes the basic problem (see chapter 11).

Chapter Fourteen

Diseases of the Aorta

Diseases of the aorta may affect the function of the heart directly or indirectly. Two congenital abnormalities affecting the left ventricle have already been discussed in chapter 11: coarctation of the aorta and supravalvular aortic stenosis. This chapter offers a brief discussion of the common acquired abnormalities of the aorta.

Atherosclerosis of the Aorta

The most important disease of the vascular system, atherosclerosis, affects the aorta as well as the smaller arteries. Yet the consequences of atherosclerotic disease in the aorta are less pronounced than in the arteries supplying blood to the heart, brain, or kidneys, which may suffer serious damage because of occlusion. Atherosclerotic changes in the intima (inner lining) of the aorta are similar to those in the intima of the smaller arteries but rarely grow large enough to interfere with the blood flow in this vessel. Changes in the aortic intima have no direct effect on its function, although atherosclerotic ulcers may become a source of thrombi, which could break loose and cause emboli in distant organs.

A special situation exists when atherosclerosis of the intima is combined with arteriosclerotic abnormalities of the aorta. The media (middle layer) of the aortic wall can then be weakened to the point that the pressure in the aorta causes a ballooning of a portion of its wall into an aneurysm.

Diseases of the Aortic Root

The aortic root—the portion of the aorta immediately above the aortic valve—and its extension, the lower part of the ascending aorta, are vulnerable to diseases other than atherosclerosis. Enlargement of the aortic root may be associated with dilatation of the ring to which aortic valve cusps are attached, thereby producing incompetence of that valve. A variety of conditions may cause abnormal dilatation of the aortic root and the lower ascending aorta— either a diffuse widening or a localized bulge (aneurysm). These include *aortitis* (inflammation of the ascending aorta), *Marfan's syndrome* (congenital weakness), and degeneration of the aorta.

Aortitis was once a common sequel of tertiary syphilis (*luetic aortitis*). Before antibiotic treatment of syphilis was discovered in the 1940s, aortic aneurysm signaled the terminal stage of that disease. Today it is rarely encountered. Aortitis is now most often associated with autoimmune diseases, such as rheumatoid arthritis, which may produce severe aortic regurgitation.

Marfan's syndrome is a hereditary condition in which the connective tissue is defective, causing structural weakness of various parts of the body. In the aorta it may produce dilatation with aortic regurgitation, aortic aneurysms, and dissection of the aorta.

Atherosclerotic changes in the aorta, as mentioned, may produce aortic aneurysms and become a source of emboli in the systemic circulation.

Aneurysms of the Aorta

Two kinds of aneurysm of the ascending aorta are shown in figure 38, saccular (b) and fusiform (c). A third type is traumatic aneurysm, an occasional sequel of "steering-wheel injury" in automobile accidents, usually affecting the descending thoracic aorta. The commonest location of degenerative aortic aneurysm affecting the elderly is the abdominal aorta. Aneurysm of the abdominal aorta generally produces no symptoms: only rarely does pain result from pressure on abdominal organs. The aneurysm, however, is of concern, for its rupture can cause sudden death due to fatal hemorrhage. Fortunately, rupture is frequently preceded by small openings in the aorta through which blood can escape, infiltrating the

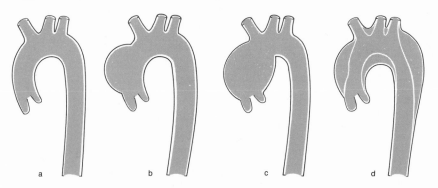

Figure 38. Diseases of the aorta. (a) Normal outline of the aorta. (b) Saccular aortic aneurysm. (c) Fusiform aortic aneurysm. (d) Dissection of the aorta.

neighboring tissue and producing symptoms; the aneurysm can then be diagnosed and surgically resected in time. The presence of abdominal aneurysms can be detected on physical examination of the abdomen in a slim person but could escape attention in someone obese. Abdominal X ray may suggest the presence of an aneurysm, which can then be outlined by ultrasound. Direct demonstration of the aneurysm by angiography is seldom needed.

Surgical resection of the aneurysm of the abdominal aorta is a common prophylactic operation. There is some controversy about the advisability of performing this operation on persons in their seventies or eighties since at that age it carries a significant risk and often requires a long hospital stay. Unless the aneurysm discovered is large, many experts suggest that its size be monitored over time and the operation performed only if growth is noticed.

Aortic dissection (also called "dissecting aneurysm") is a dangerous condition that can lead to catastrophic emergencies. Dissection means separation of the inner and outer layers of the aorta produced by a tear in the intima; blood can then enter the space between the layers and widen it into a channel (see figure 38d). Blood can flow through the artifical channel parallel to the normal lumen of the aorta and reenter the latter through an exit tear. Once considered a specific disease caused by genetic cystic degeneration of the aortic media, it is now accepted that aortic dissection may be due to the aging process alone. The usual underlying factor for aortic dissection is hypertension.

Various types of dissection are recognized. The tear may develop in the aortic root and affect only the ascending aorta, with the exit channel in the aortic arch. Another type of dissection involves the entire length of the aorta, with the entry tear in the aortic root and the exit tear in the abdominal aorta, producing a double-lumen aorta. A third type of dissection affects the descending thoracic aorta communicating with the abdominal aorta. This variety may be part of traumatic aortic aneurysm.

The principal danger of aortic dissection is rupture of the rather weak outer wall of the new channel and fatal hemorrhage. Dissection of the ascending aorta has some specific consequences. The artificial channel, in which blood is under high pressure (equal to that in the aorta), may constrict the exit of arterial branches of the aorta, producing decreased blood flow to the head and upper extremities. Furthermore, dissection of the aortic root above the aortic valve may distort the aortic orifice to a point that the normal aortic leaflets can no longer close tightly during diastole; hence, severe acute aortic regurgitation may develop. Occlusion of arterial branches of the aorta from the dissection may include coronary arteries, producing myocardial infarction, or the carotid artery, producing stroke.

The abrupt onset of a tear in the aorta is almost always associated with severe pain in the chest, yet the condition must not be mistaken for myocardial infarction. Even though myocardial infarction is a hundred times more common than aortic dissection, the medical team in an emergency unit must be able to distinguish them if proper lifesaving treatment is to be administered. Since the size of the new channel is related to the elasticity of the adventitia (outer layer) of the aorta, sometimes the channel is narrow, the outer wall firm, and the consequences minimal. The initial chest pain may be ignored or misdiagnosed, and the condition may remain unrecognized until much later (as "chronic" dissection of the aorta).

Treatment of aortic dissection consists of medical management or surgical resection of the dissected portion of the aorta and its replacement with a synthetic graft. This heroic operation carries a high risk; nonetheless, it has been performed in certain cardiac treatment centers with reasonable success. The timing of the operation varies: immediate surgery is indicated if serious consequences of the dissection are in evidence. Medical treatment may include the use of drugs to reduce blood pressure and decrease the force with which the blood is ejected into the aorta.

Glossary

Addison's disease.   A disease caused by destruction of the adrenal glands, characterized by weakness, low blood pressure, and brown pigmentation of the skin.

Adventitia.   The outer layer of an artery.

Aldosterone.   A hormone of the cortex (outer part) of the adrenal gland, regulating salt and water balance in body tissues.

Alveolus.   The terminal air sac in the lungs, into which blood from the capillaries deposits carbon dioxide and from which oxygen is extracted.

Amyloidosis.   A disease in which an abnormal protein substance, amyloid, is deposited in various tissues, including the heart.

Aneurysm.   An abnormal outpouching of a wall of the heart or a blood vessel (particularly the aorta).

Angiocardiography.   Visualization of the contents of the heart or blood vessels by injecting a contrast liquid into the bloodstream and recording the X-ray image.

Angiography.   Contrast visualization of the blood vessels only. See also *angiocardiography.*

Angioplasty.   A catheter procedure on blood vessels, using a balloon or other special device. See also *balloon angioplasty.*

Angiotensin.   One of the hormones regulating blood pressure.

Anticoagulant.   A drug or agent interfering with the clotting of blood.

Aortic valve.   See *semilunar valves.*

Arrhythmia.   A general term for various disturbances of the rhythm or rate of the heartbeat.

Arteriography.   Contrast visualization of the arteries only. See also *angiocardiography.*

Arteriole.   The smallest-caliber vessel of the arterial system, which plays an important role in regulating blood pressure.

Arteriosclerosis.   "Hardening of the arteries," a broad term referring to degenerative, age-related diseases of the arteries.

Ascites.   Abnormal accumulation of serous fluid in the abdominal cavity.

Asymptomatic.   Showing no symptoms from an existing disease.

Atherosclerosis.   A disease of the arteries affecting the intima and tending to narrow the vessels.

Atrioventricular.   Located at the junction between the atria and the ventricles of the heart.

Atrioventricular block.   Disturbance of the conduction of impulses from atrium to ventricle of the heart.

Atrioventricular node.   Small structure through which impulses are conducted from atrium to ventricle.

Atrioventricular valves.   The *mitral valve* (left side) and *tricuspid valve* (right side), separating the atria from the ventricles.

Auscultation.   The act of listening to the sound of the heart, lungs, or other organs, usually with the aid of a stethoscope.

Autonomic.   Self-regulating.

Autonomic nervous system.   A system of nerves controlling the function of the heart, blood vessels, and certain other organs.

A-V.   Atrioventricular (node or block).

Balloon angioplasty.   A procedure for dilating a stenotic blood vessel by inflating a balloon at the end of a catheter.

Balloon valvuloplasty.   A procedure for dilating a stenotic valve by inflating a balloon at the end of a catheter.

Block (in reference to the conduction of cardiac impulses).   Interruption or delay in the conductive pathway.

Bradycardia.   Abnormally slow heartbeat.

Bundle branch.   One of the two divisions of the bundle of His.

Bundle of His.   The part of the cardiac conductive system transmitting impulses from the atrio-ventricular node to the ventricles.

Calcific.   Containing deposits of calcium.

Capillary.   The thinnest of the blood vessels, through which oxygen is supplied to tissues.

Cardiogenic.   Related to or caused by the heart (such as cardiogenic shock).

Carditis.   An inflammatory disease of the heart involving all three of its layers.

Cardioversion.   The administration of electric shock to the chest to treat certain arrhythmias.

Catheterization (pertaining to the heart).   Diagnostic tests involving the insertion of a catheter into the vascular system.

Chordae tendineae.   Cordlike structures connecting the edges of the mitral valve with the papillary muscles.

Collateral circulation.   Arteries or veins providing detours for supplying blood to a portion of an organ in which the normal channels are blocked or narrowed.

Commissure (in cardiac valves).   The junction or the free space between leaflets of a valve.

Congestion.   Excessive accumulation of blood in an organ or part of the body.

Coronary.   Pertaining to the blood supply to the heart itself.

Corticosteroid.   A hormone produced by the adrenal cortex or its synthetic equivalent.

Cushing's disease (or *syndrome*).   A disease caused by malfunction of the pituitary gland or adrenal gland, characterized by obesity and high blood pressure.

Cyanosis.   A bluish coloration of the skin, especially visible in the lips and fingertips, due to reduced oxygen content in blood vessels near the surface.

Depolarization.   The discharge of electrical potential by heart muscle cells just before contraction.

Diastole. The stage of the heart cycle comprising the entire period of relaxation of the heart muscle.

Dissection of the aorta (or *dissecting aneurysm*). Separation of the layers of the aorta, permitting the blood to create a second, abnormal channel.

Dissociation (in arrhythmias). Abnormal, independent electrical activity of the atria and the ventricles.

Diuretic. A drug increasing the flow of urine.

Dyspnea. Abnormal shortness of breath.

Eclampsia. Convulsions occurring in pregnant women with hypertension.

Ectopic (pertaining to cardiac rhythm). Originating from a source other than the normal pacemaker.

Edema. Abnormal accumulation of fluid in the body, usually manifested as swelling of the ankles or other parts of the body.

Effusion. Accumulation of fluid in a body cavity, such as the chest (pleural effusion) or pericardum.

Electrolyte. A chemical substance in ionic form in solution capable of conducting electricity, such as sodium, potassium, or calcium.

Electrophysiology. The study of the electrical activity of an organ.

Embolus. A plug of abnormal material (usually a clot) obstructing blood flow in an artery, transported by the bloodstream from another part of the circulation.

Endocardium. The inner lining of the heart.

Enzyme. A protein capable of accelerating certain chemical reactions.

Epicardium. The outer lining of the heart; one of the two layers of the pericardium.

Extrasystole. A heartbeat occurring out of the normal sequence.

Fibrillation. Uncoordinated twitching of the heart muscle, replacing the normal beating sequence and causing heart failure.

Flutter. Abnormally rapid contraction of the atria or ventricles, reducing or eliminating the function of the affected chamber.

Glomerulonephritis. Inflammatory disease of the kidneys, often producing hypertension.

Gradient. A difference in pressure between two adjacent points of the circulation.

Hemodynamics. The dynamics of movement of the blood in the body.

Hemosiderosis. A condition associated with abnormal iron storage in various organs.

Hydrostatic pressure. Pressure exerted within a blood vessel in relation to other structures.

Hypercholesterolemia. An abnormally high level of cholesterol in the blood.

Hyperlipidemia. An abnormally high level of fat in the blood.

Hypertrophy. Excessive growth of a muscle or an organ.

Insufficiency, valvular. See *regurgitation, valvular.*

Intima. The inner layer of the wall of an artery.

Invasive (pertaining to a test or other procedure). Involving introduction of an instrument into the body.

Ischemia. Local deficiency of blood supply due to obstruction or spasm of the supplying artery.

Isometric. Referring to change in the tension of a muscle without a corresponding change in its size (such as isometric contraction and relaxation of the heart muscle).

Junctional (pertaining to cardiac rhythm). Originating at the junction between the A-V node and the bundle of His. *Junctional rhythm* is also referred to as *A-V nodal rhythm.*

Lipoprotein. A chemical substance in the blood combining proteins and fats.

Lumen. The cavity inside a tubular organ, such as an artery.

Media. The middle layer of a blood vessel.

Mitral valve. See *atrioventricular valves.*

Monitor (in the management of heart disease). Continuous visual display or record of an electrocardiographic lead, pressure curve, or other circulatory modality.

Murmur. An abnormal auscultatory sound originating in the heart and indicating turbulent blood flow.

Myocarditis.   Inflammatory disease of the heart muscle.

Myocardium.   The muscular layer of the heart; the heart muscle.

Node.   A part of the conducting system. See *atrioventricular node, sinoatrial node.*

Oscilloscope.   An instrument capable of displaying electrical impulses on a screen, used in electrocardiographic monitoring, echocardiography, and X-ray imaging.

Osmotic pressure.   The pressure in a liquid exerted by substances dissolved in it.

Output, cardiac.   The quantity of blood ejected by a cardiac ventricle in one minute.

Overload, cardiac.   Increased work demands on the heart.

Pacemaker.   (1) A group of cells in which rhythmic impulses governing heart actions are generated. (2) An electronic apparatus connected to the heart and inducing its rhythmic stimulation.

Pacing.   Using an electronic pacemaker.

Papillary muscles.   Two cone-shaped muscles arising from the apex of each cardiac ventricle, to which the *chordae tendineae* are attached.

Paroxysm.   A sudden attack involving change from a normal to an abnormal state in a body function.

Percutaneous.   Introducing an instrument into the body through the intact skin.

Pericardium.   The outer coating of the heart, consisting of an inner membrane firmly attached to the heart (*epicardium*) and an outer one forming a loose sack (*parietal pericardium*).

Placebo.   An inactive substance (such as sugar) placed in a tablet or capsule, used as a control in drug testing.

Pleura.   The outer lining of the lungs.

Polycystic disease.   A condition producing multiple cysts in various organs, frequently affecting the kidneys.

Prolapse (of the mitral valve).   Abnormal displacement of a portion of a mitral-valve cusp during systole.

Prophylactic.   Preventive.

Pulmonary.   Relating to the lungs.

Pulmonary circulation.   The smaller of the two circuits, in which blood ejected by the right ventricle is sent to the lungs before returning to the left atrium; also called the lesser circulation.

Pulmonary valve.   See *semilunar valves.*

Pyelonephritis.   An inflammatory disease of the portion of the kidneys that excretes urine.

Radiography.   The procedure of recording X-ray images on film.

Reentry (in arrhythmias).   Reactivation of the heart from a single impulse.

Regurgitation, valvular.   Faulty function of a cardiac valve permitting backflow of blood.

Renin.   A hormone produced by the kidney involved in regulating blood pressure.

Renal.   Relating to the kidneys.

S-A.   Sinoatrial (node).

Sarcoidosis.   A chronic disease of unknown origin characterized by the formation of small nodules in various organs including the heart.

Septum, cardiac.   The partition between the two sides of the heart, consisting of the atrial septum and the ventricular septum.

Semilunar valves.   Either of the two outflow valves from the heart, the pulmonary valve (right side) and the aortic valve (left side).

Shunt.   Blood flow through an abnormal connection between the two sides of the heart or between various vascular structures.

Standstill, cardiac.   Absence of contraction of the atria or the ventricles due to failure of the electrical impulse to arrive, or failure to respond to the impulse.

Sinoatrial node.   Uppermost part of the cardiac conduction system; the normally active pacemaker.

Stenosis.   A narrowing of the diameter of any structure through which a liquid is conducted, including arteries and cardiac valves.

Sign (in diagnosis).   An abnormality detected objectively by the physician (as opposed to a symptom).

Stroke volume.   The quantity of blood ejected by each ventricle in a single contraction.

Supraventricular (pertaining to an abnormal cardiac rhythm).   Originating in the atrium or the atrioventricular node.

Symptom.   A subjective manifestation of disease felt or observed by the patient.

Syndrome.   A group of signs and symptoms occurring together but not as well defined as a disease.

Systemic circulation.   The larger of the two circuits, in which blood ejected by the left ventricle supplies most of the body before returning to the right atrium; also called the greater circulation.

Systole.   The stage of the heart cycle involving muscular contraction.

Tamponade, pericardial.   Excessive fluid in the pericardium interfering with cardiac action.

Tachycardia.   Rapid heartbeat, usually defined as 100 beats a minute or more.

Therapy.   Treatment.

Thrombosis.   The process of intravascular clot formation.

Thrombus.   A clot formed inside a blood vessel.

Tricuspid valve.   See *atrioventricular valves.*

Valvotomy.   Surgery on a cardiac valve to relieve valvular stenosis.

Valvuloplasty.   Repair of a valvular abnormality either by surgery or by manipulation of a balloon-equipped cardiac catheter.

Ventriculography.   Contrast visualization of the ventricle to observe its function.

Vegetation.   A small wartlike structure developing on heart valves in infective endocarditis.

Vena cava.   One of the two large veins (superior and inferior) entering the right atrium and returning blood to the heart.

Index

(Italicized page numbers indicate figures.)

Compositor: Huron Valley Graphics
Printer: Malloy Lithographing, Inc.
Binder: John H. Dekker & Sons
Text: 11/13 Caledonia
Display: Caledonia